Handbook of
Arthroscopy

Handbook of Arthroscopy

Editors

Sachin Yashwant Kale
MBBS MS(Orthopedics) FCPS DOrtho
Fellowship in Arthroplasty
President NMOA, EC Member BOS
Professor and Head
DY Patil University School of Medicine
Apollo Hospital, Belapur
Fortis Hiranandani Hospital, Vashi
Navi Mumbai, Maharashtra, India

Rohit Mahesh Sane
MBBS MD(Pharmacology) MS(Orthopedics)
DFM(FIFA) FASM(India)
Orthopedic Sports Medicine Surgeon and
AOA Shoulder Surgery Fellow (Australia)
Department of Shoulder Surgery
Australian Shoulder Research Institute
Brisbane, Australia

Co-Editors

Prasad Liladhar Chaudhari
MBBS MS(Orthopedics)
DNB(Orthopedics) DOrtho FCPS
FSES(SK)
Professor, Department of
Orthopedics
DY Patil University School of Medicine
Navi Mumbai, Maharashtra, India

Bhushan Jaywantrao Patil
MBBS DNB(Orthopedics) DOrtho
FASM(Singapore)
Professor and Head
Department of Sport Medicine
DY Patil University School of Medicine
Navi Mumbai, Maharashtra, India

Sandeep Narayan Deore MBBS
MS(Orthopedics)
Professor
Department of Orthopedics
DY Patil University School of
Medicine
Navi Mumbai, Maharashtra, India

Pramod Bhor MBBS
MS(Orthopedics)
Director
Department of Orthopedics
Fortis Hiranandani
Navi Mumbai, Maharashtra, India

Aditya R Gunjotikar MBBS
MS(Orthopedics) FASM
Assistant Professor
Department of Orthopedics
DY Patil University School of Medicine
Navi Mumbai, Maharashtra, India

Vaibhav J Koli MBBS
MS(Orthopedics) FAA
Assistant Professor
Department of Orthopedics
DY Patil University School of Medicine
Navi Mumbai, Maharashtra, India

Rahul V Davari MBBS MS(Orthopedics)
Assistant Professor
Department of Orthopedics
Terna Medical College and Hospital, Vashi
Fortis Hiranandani Hospital
Kokilaben Dhirubhai Ambani Hospital
Medicity Hospital, Kharghar
Acharya Shri Nanesh Hospital, Belapur
Navi Mumbai, Maharashtra, India

Foreword

Nicholas Antao

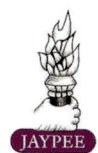

JAYPEE BROTHERS MEDICAL PUBLISHERS
The Health Sciences Publisher
New Delhi | London

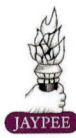 **Jaypee Brothers Medical Publishers (P) Ltd**

Headquarters
EMCA House
23/23-B, Ansari Road, Daryaganj
New Delhi 110 002, India
Landline: +91-11-23272143, +91-11-23272703
+91-11-23282021, +91-11-23245672
E-mail: jaypee@jaypeebrothers.com

Corporate Office
Jaypee Brothers Medical Publishers (P) Ltd.
4838/24, Ansari Road, Daryaganj
New Delhi 110 002, India
Phone: +91-11-43574357
Fax: +91-11-43574314
E-mail: jaypee@jaypeebrothers.com

Overseas Office
JP Medical Ltd.
83, Victoria Street, London
SW1H 0HW (UK)
Phone: +44-20 3170 8910
Fax: +44(0)20 3008 6180
E-mail: info@jpmedpub.com

Website: www.jaypeebrothers.com
Website: www.jaypeedigital.com

© 2025, Jaypee Brothers Medical Publishers

The views and opinions expressed in this book are solely those of the original contributor(s)/author(s) and do not necessarily represent those of editor(s) or publisher of the book.

All rights reserved. No part of this publication may be reproduced, stored or transmitted in any form or by any means, electronic, mechanical, photocopying, recording or otherwise, without the prior permission in writing of the publishers.

All brand names and product names used in this book are trade names, service marks, trademarks or registered trademarks of their respective owners. The publisher is not associated with any product or vendor mentioned in this book.

Medical knowledge and practice change constantly. This book is designed to provide accurate, authoritative information about the subject matter in question. However, readers are advised to check the most current information available on procedures included and check information from the manufacturer of each product to be administered, to verify the recommended dose, formula, method and duration of administration, adverse effects and contraindications. It is the responsibility of the practitioner to take all appropriate safety precautions. Neither the publisher nor the author(s)/editor(s) assume any liability for any injury and/or damage to persons or property arising from or related to use of material in this book.

This book is sold on the understanding that the publisher is not engaged in providing professional medical services. If such advice or services are required, the services of a competent medical professional should be sought.

Every effort has been made where necessary to contact holders of copyright to obtain permission to reproduce copyright material. If any have been inadvertently overlooked, the publisher will be pleased to make the necessary arrangements at the first opportunity.

Inquiries for bulk sales may be solicited at: jaypee@jaypeebrothers.com

Handbook of Arthroscopy / Sachin Yashwant Kale, Rohit Mahesh Sane
First Edition: **2025**
ISBN: 978-93-6616-701-5
Printed at: Samrat Offset Pvt. Ltd.

Dedication

This book is dedicated to all those who have been a part of my journey—those who have taught me, supported me, and inspired me to strive for excellence in the field of orthopedic surgery.

To my family:

To my beloved spouse, Dr Smruti. Your unwavering love, patience, and encouragement have been my anchor through every challenge. Your quiet strength and belief in me have provided the foundation upon which I stand today. Without your support, this book would not have been possible.

To my wonderful daughters, Sachiti and Saanvi. Your curiosity, boundless energy, and enthusiasm for life remind me every day why the pursuit of knowledge is so valuable. You are my inspiration, my pride, and my greatest joy.

To my parents, Yashwant Kale and Sulochana Kale, and my in-laws, Ramesh Parate and Pramila Parate, who have instilled in me the values of hard work, perseverance, and integrity. Your blessings, sacrifices, and wisdom have shaped me into the person and professional I am today.

To my mentors and teachers:

I owe a deep debt of gratitude to my mentors and teachers, whose wisdom, guidance, and encouragement have shaped my understanding of orthopedic surgery. Their dedication to teaching and patient care has been an inspiration throughout my career. In particular, I am profoundly grateful to those who have guided me through the intricacies of arthroscopic surgery, sharing their insights, experiences, and invaluable lessons along the way.

To my co-editor and esteemed contributors:

To my co-editor, Dr Rohit Mahesh Sane. Thank you for your unwavering dedication, expertise, and collaborative spirit. Your contributions to this book have been invaluable, and your knowledge in orthopedic sports medicine and arthroscopy has played a crucial role in shaping this work. Your meticulous approach, innovative mindset, and deep passion for advancing arthroscopic surgery are truly commendable.

To all the contributing authors. This book is as much yours as it is mine. Each of you has brought your unique experiences, perspectives, and expertise to this project, making it a rich and comprehensive resource for the next generation of orthopedic surgeons. Your hard work, commitment, and willingness to share your knowledge will undoubtedly leave a lasting impact on the field of arthroscopy.

To my colleagues and friends:

To my colleagues and friends in the orthopedic and medical communities. Thank you for your camaraderie, support, and intellectual stimulation. Our discussions, debates, and shared experiences have shaped my professional journey and strengthened my resolve to contribute meaningfully to our field.

To my patients:

To the patients who have entrusted me with their care. You are my greatest teachers. Your resilience, trust, and unwavering faith in the healing process inspire me every day. This book is dedicated to you and to the countless individuals whose lives are touched by orthopedic surgery.

To the future generations of orthopedic surgeons:

Finally, this book is dedicated to the residents, fellows, and young orthopedic surgeons who aspire to master arthroscopy and push the boundaries of surgical excellence. May this handbook serve as a guide, a source of knowledge, and a tool to enhance your skills and confidence. The future of orthopedic surgery lies in your hands, and I hope this book helps you in your journey to becoming skilled, compassionate, and innovative surgeons.

With deepest respect, gratitude, and dedication!

Sachin Yashwant Kale

Contributors

Aditya R Gunjotikar MBBS MS(Orthopedics) FASM
Assistant Professor
Department of Orthopedics
DY Patil University School of Medicine
Navi Mumbai, Maharashtra, India

Arvind J Vatkar MBBS MS(Orthopedics) AFIH MCh(Spine Surgery) Advanced Spine Surgery Fellowship(UK)
Assistant Professor
Department of Orthopedics
MGM Medical College
Navi Mumbai, Maharashtra, India

Col Anup Krishnan MBBS DSM PhD
Director and Professor
Department of Sports and Exercise Medicine
School of Sports, Exercise and Nutrition Sciences, DY Patil University
Navi Mumbai, Maharashtra, India

Bhushan Jaywantrao Patil MBBS DNB(Orthopedics) DOrtho FASM(Singapore)
Professor and Head
Department of Sport Medicine
DY Patil University School of Medicine
Navi Mumbai, Maharashtra, India

Gaurav Kanade MBBS MS(Orthopedics)
Fellowship in Arthroplasty
Associate Professor
Department of Orthopedics
DY Patil University School of Medicine
Navi Mumbai, Maharashtra, India

Prakash D Samant MBBS MS(Orthopedics)
Professor and Head
Department of Orthopedics
DY Patil University School of Medicine
Navi Mumbai, Maharashtra, India

Pramod Bhor MBBS MS(Orthopedics)
Director
Department of Orthopedics
Fortis Hiranandani
Navi Mumbai, Maharashtra, India

Prasad Liladhar Chaudhari MBBS MS(Orthopedics) DNB(Orthopedics) DOrtho FCPS FSES(SK)
Professor
Department of Orthopedics
DY Patil University School of Medicine
Navi Mumbai, Maharashtra, India

Prerna Pradeep Ghodke BPT
MPT(Physiotherapy in Neurosciences)
Assistant Professor
Department of Musculoskeletal Physiotherapy
School of Physiotherapy, DY Patil University
Navi Mumbai, Maharashtra, India

Rahul V Davari MBBS MS(Orthopedics)
Assistant Professor
Department of Orthopedics
Terna Medical College and Hospital, Vashi
Fortis Hiranandani Hospital
Kokilaben Dhirubhai Ambani Hospital
Medicity Hospital, Kharghar
Acharya Shri Nanesh Hospital, Belapur
Navi Mumbai, Maharashtra, India

Rohit Mahesh Sane MBBS
MD(Pharmacology) MS(Orthopedics)
DFM(FIFA) FASM(India)
Orthopedic Sports Medicine Surgeon and AOA Shoulder Surgery Fellow (Australia)
Department of Shoulder Surgery
Australian Shoulder Research Institute
Brisbane, Australia

Contributors

Sachin Yashwant Kale MBBS
MS(Orthopedics) FCPS DOrtho Fellowship in Arthroplasty
President NMOA, EC Member BOS
Professor and Head
Department of Orthopedics
DY Patil University School of Medicine
Apollo Hospital, Belapur
Fortis Hiranandani Hospital, Vashi
Navi Mumbai, Maharashtra, India

Sachiti Sachin Kale MBBS (Second Year)
Lokmanya Tilak Medical College and Sion Hospital
Mumbai, Maharashtra, India

Sagar Subhash Deshpande BPT
MPT(Physiotherapy in Neurosciences)
Associate Professor
Department of Neurophysiotherapy
School of Physiotherapy, DY Patil University
Navi Mumbai, Maharashtra, India

Sandeep Narayan Deore MBBS
MS(Orthopedics)
Professor
Department of Orthopedics
DY Patil University School of Medicine
Navi Mumbai, Maharashtra, India

Sanjay B Dhar MBBS MS(Orthopedics)
DNB(Orthopedics)
Professor and Head
Department of Orthopedics
DY Patil University School of Medicine
Navi Mumbai, Maharashtra, India

Shikhar D Singh MBBS MS(Orthopedics)
Associate Professor
Department of Orthopedics
DY Patil University School of Medicine
Navi Mumbai, Maharashtra, India

Shivam Mehra MBBS MS(Orthopedics)
Short-term Fellowship in Deformity Correction and Limb Lengthening Surgeries
Consultant
Department of Orthopedics
Mehra Hospital and Research Institute
Lucknow, Uttar Pradesh, India

Sunil H Shetty MBBS MS(Orthopedics)
CCCR PGDHHM
Professor and Head
Department of Orthopedics
DY Patil University School of Medicine
Navi Mumbai, Maharashtra, India

Sushmit Singh MBBS MS(Orthopedics)
MRCS
Trauma and Orthopedics Registrar
Department of Orthopedics
Warrington and Halton, NHS Teaching Hospital
Warrington, United Kingdom

Vaibhav J Koli MBBS MS(Orthopedics) FAA
Assistant Professor
Department of Orthopedics
DY Patil University School of Medicine
Navi Mumbai, Maharashtra, India

Vishal Kumar MBBS MS(Orthopedics)
DNB(Orthopedics) FRCS
Adjunct Professor
Department of Orthopedics
PGIMER
Chandigarh, India

Foreword

I feel honored and privileged to write the foreword for *Handbook of Arthroscopy* by the members of the Bombay Orthopaedic Society (BOS), headed by Dr Sachin Yashwant Kale.

BOS has been at the forefront, pioneering and leading the dissemination of arthroscopy knowledge in India.

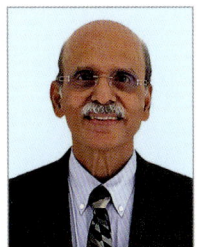

The first international exposure to arthroscopy in Mumbai occurred in 1978, thanks to the efforts of the late Dr Pravin Vora, who was the Secretary of the Indian Arthroscopy Society (IAS) at the time. Dr Dinesh Patel from New York played a key role in bringing together an excellent foreign faculty to exchange and share knowledge on arthroscopy through didactic lectures and hands-on dry bone workshops. Following this international conference and workshop, Dr Abhay Narvekar and I initiated dry and cadaveric workshops and live demonstrations at various institutions in Bombay. These events were organized under the aegis of BOS when I served as the Secretary of the Society. Delegates were provided with xerox-printed booklets of the lectures, and over time, the cadaveric workshops became a regular annual feature on the calendars of both BOS and the IAS.

The expansion of arthroscopy workshops continued with the support of the industry. At the Indian Arthroscopy Conference in Bombay, we hosted the first ISAKOS (International Society of Arthroscopy, Knee Surgery, and Orthopaedic Sports Medicine) sponsored hands-on cadaveric workshop in India, with foreign faculty member Dr Ramon Cugat from Barcelona. This was organized under the leadership of Dr Anant Joshi, with Dr Dinshaw Pardiwalla as the scientific chairman and myself as the Secretary of the IAS Conference, held at Seth GS Medical College and KEM Hospital in 1984.

ISAKOS subsequently sponsored many such workshops and training initiatives for arthroscopy in India. Later, Dr Gopalkrishnan SG, through IAS, initiated fellowships to help numerous students from across India travel and learn from established arthroscopy centers.

Since the cadaveric workshops have become a regular feature in India, the need for a comprehensive handbook on basic arthroscopy has become evident. This book will undoubtedly be a great resource for young students eager to specialize in arthroscopy.

The publication of the *Handbook of Arthroscopy* is a significant effort by Dr Sachin Yashwant Kale and his team of authors. They have devoted tremendous effort and dedication to compiling this valuable resource, which, I am told, marks the beginning of a series of such handbooks to be published in the future.

I am hopeful and confident that more young authors will contribute to this endeavor in the near future, providing guidance to young orthopedic surgeons and greatly enhancing their learning process as they explore the basics of arthroscopy.

Nicholas Antao MS FCPS DNB(Orthopedics)
Consultant Orthopedics
Traumatology, Arthroscopy and Sports Medicine and
Joint Replacement Surgeon
Past-President of BOS
Past President of IAS
Mumbai, Maharashtra, India

Preface

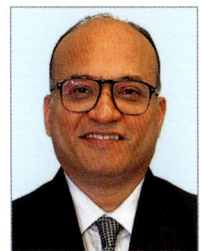

Sachin Yashwant Kale

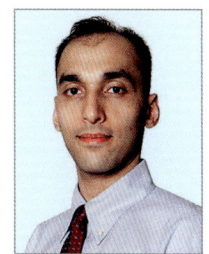

Rohit Mahesh Sane

Arthroscopy has revolutionized orthopedic surgery, offering minimally invasive solutions for diagnosing and treating a wide range of joint disorders. With advancements in technology and surgical techniques, arthroscopy has become an indispensable tool in modern orthopedic practice. This handbook aims to serve as a comprehensive yet concise guide for orthopedic surgeons, residents, and fellows seeking to deepen their understanding and refine their skills in arthroscopy.

The *"Handbook of Arthroscopy"* is designed to provide both foundational knowledge and practical insights into the evolving field of arthroscopic surgery. Covering key topics such as knee and shoulder arthroscopy, graft selection, ligament reconstructions, and rehabilitation, this book offers a structured approach to the essential concepts and techniques required for successful arthroscopic procedures. Each chapter is written by experienced surgeons and specialists in the field, ensuring that the content is evidence-based, clinically relevant, and easy to apply in practice.

The book is structured to facilitate quick reference, with step-by-step explanations of surgical procedures, illustrations, and case-based discussions. Special attention has been given to aspects such as patient positioning, portal placements, and postsurgical rehabilitation, which are critical for optimal patient outcomes. Additionally, we have included a dedicated section on the psychology of an arthroscopic surgeon, recognizing the mental resilience and decision-making skills required in this demanding field.

We extend our gratitude to all the contributors whose expertise and dedication have made this handbook possible. Their collective experience and knowledge will undoubtedly benefit readers who wish to enhance their proficiency in arthroscopic surgery. We also acknowledge the patients, mentors, and colleagues who continue to inspire us in our pursuit of excellence.

We hope this handbook serves as a valuable resource, equipping orthopedic surgeons with the confidence and competence to perform arthroscopic procedures effectively and improve patient care.

Acknowledgments

Writing this book has been an extraordinary journey, and I am deeply grateful to all those who have supported and inspired me along the way.

First and foremost, I want to express my heartfelt gratitude to my family—to my spouse, Dr Smruti, whose unwavering support, patience, and encouragement have been my anchor throughout this project, and to my daughters, Sachiti and Saanvi, whose curiosity and love have been my constant source of motivation. Their belief in me has made this achievement possible.

I am profoundly thankful to my co-editor, Dr Rohit Mahesh Sane, for his invaluable contributions, expertise, and unwavering commitment to making this handbook a comprehensive resource. His deep knowledge in orthopedic sports medicine and arthroscopy, coupled with his dedication to academic excellence, has been instrumental in shaping this work.

I extend my sincere appreciation to all the authors who have contributed their expertise to this book: Drs Arvind J Vatkar, Shivam Mehra, Aditya R Gunjotikar, Vaibhav J Koli, Prakash D Samant, Sandeep Narayan Deore, Shikhar D Singh, Sanjay B Dhar, Vishal Kumar, Prasad Liladhar Chaudhari, Gaurav Kanade, Bhushan Jaywantrao Patil, Sushmit Singh, Pramod Bhor, Rahul V Davari, Sunil H Shetty, Anup Krishnan, Sagar Subhash Deshpande, Prerna Pradeep Ghodke, and many more whose collective efforts have made this book a rich source of knowledge. Their willingness to share their experience and insights has been fundamental in creating this resource for our fellow orthopedic professionals.

I also extend my gratitude to my editors, whose keen insights, meticulous attention to detail, and thoughtful feedback have significantly improved this work. Their guidance and expertise have been invaluable in ensuring the clarity and accuracy of the content.

I would like to acknowledge my publisher, Jaypee Brothers Medical Publishers, for believing in this book and providing the resources and platform to bring it to life. Their professionalism and commitment have been essential in realizing this dream.

I am deeply grateful to my mentors, colleagues, and peers in the medical and academic communities. Their thought-provoking discussions, research support, and encouragement have played a pivotal role in enriching this book.

A special note of appreciation goes to the patients whose experiences have shaped this book. Their stories remind us of the importance of continuous learning and improvement in orthopedic surgery.

Finally, I want to thank my readers. Their interest and engagement inspire me to continue exploring and sharing knowledge. I hope this book serves as a valuable resource and guide in their professional journey.

Thank you all for being a part of this journey!

Sachin Yashwant Kale

Contents

1. **Introduction to Arthroscopy** — 1
   Rohit Mahesh Sane, Sachin Yashwant Kale, Arvind J Vatkar, Shivam Mehra

2. **Knee Positioning, Draping, and Portals** — 11
   Aditya R Gunjotikar, Vaibhav J Koli, Sachin Yashwant Kale, Prakash D Samant

3. **Grafts** — 23
   Sandeep Narayan Deore, Rohit Mahesh Sane, Shikhar D Singh, Sanjay B Dhar, Sachin Yashwant Kale

4. **Diagnostic Round (Knee), Indications, and Contraindications** — 37
   Vaibhav J Koli, Vishal Kumar, Sachin Yashwant Kale, Rohit Mahesh Sane

5. **Anterior Cruciate Ligament** — 45
   Aditya R Gunjotikar, Rohit Mahesh Sane, Prasad Liladhar Chaudhari, Gaurav Kanade

6. **Meniscus** — 58
   Bhushan Jaywantrao Patil, Sandeep Narayan Deore, Prasad Liladhar Chaudhari, Sushmit Singh

7. **Posterior Cruciate Ligament** — 69
   Bhushan Jaywantrao Patil, Sandeep Narayan Deore, Sachin Yashwant Kale, Pramod Bhor

8. **Shoulder Positioning, Draping, and Portals** — 75
   Pramod Bhor, Rahul V Davari, Sachin Yashwant Kale, Rohit Mahesh Sane

9. **Diagnostic Round (Shoulder), Indications and Complications** — 87
   Prasad Liladhar Chaudhari, Rohit Mahesh Sane, Sandeep Narayan Deore, Sachin Yashwant Kale

10. **Rotator Cuff** — 92
    Sandeep Narayan Deore, Pramod Bhor, Sunil H Shetty, Sachin Yashwant Kale

11. **Anterior Instability** — 104
    Vaibhav J Koli, Aditya R Gunjotikar, Rohit Mahesh Sane, Shivam Mehra

12. **Frozen Shoulder**   126
   Sachin Yashwant Kale, Anup Krishnan, Arvind J Vatkar, Aditya R Gunjotikar, Vishal Kumar

13. **The Psychology of an Arthroscopy Surgeon**   132
   Bhushan Jaywantrao Patil, Anup Krishnan, Sachin Yashwant Kale, Pramod Bhor, Sachiti Sachin Kale

14. **Rehabilitation in Knee Ligament Arthroscopic Surgeries**   139
   Sagar Subhash Deshpande, Prerna Pradeep Ghodke, Sachin Yashwant Kale

15. **Rehabilitation in Arthroscopic Rotator Cuff Repair and Capsular Release in Frozen Shoulder**   150
   Sagar Subhash Deshpande, Prerna Pradeep Ghodke, Sachin Yashwant Kale

Author Publications   165

Index   167

CHAPTER 1

Introduction to Arthroscopy

Rohit Mahesh Sane, Sachin Yashwant Kale,
Arvind J Vatkar, Shivam Mehra

■ ARTHROSCOPE AND LENS

The arthroscope (telescope) is the main equipment of the arthroscopic system. It comprises an eyepiece, a light cable attachment, multiple lenses, and optical fibers for transmitting light into the joint **(Fig. 1)**. The lenses, fiberoptics, and metal casing constitute the arthroscope barrel.

Modern arthroscopes are based on the Hopkins rod lens system, which combines a smaller overall diameter with a substantially larger visual field and a brighter image **(Fig. 2)**. The main factors to be considered in selecting an arthroscope are viewing angle, barrel length, coupling mechanism, diameter, image quality, and sterilizability.

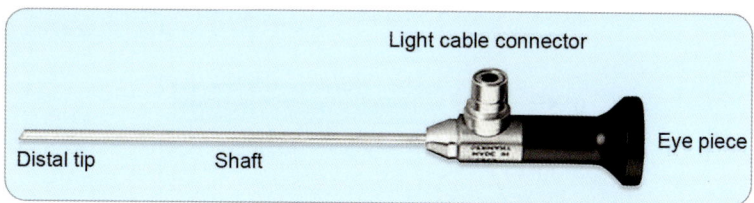

FIG. 1: Parts of a scope.

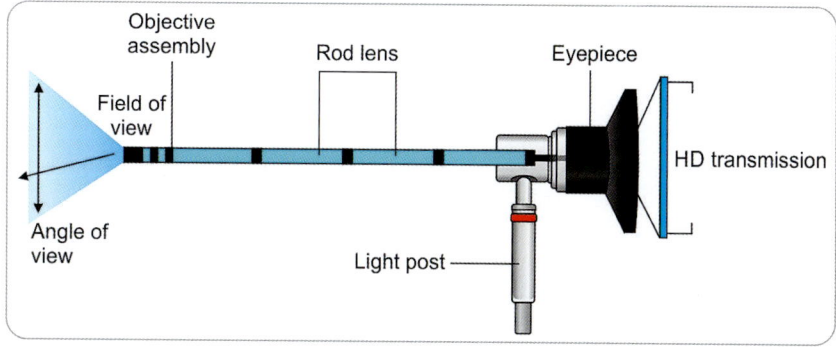

FIG. 2: Arthroscopic lens.

Viewing Angle

Arthroscopes are available with various view angles: 0° (forward-view scope), 30° wide-angle, and 70° wide-angle. In a 0° arthroscope, the visual field is directly in line with the barrel axis. The scope itself must be angled in order to change the field of view, and it can be advanced or retracted to narrow or widen the image. Rotating the scope does not affect the view.

In a 30° arthroscope, the viewing angle is directed 30° relative to the optical axis (barrel axis) of the scope. Wide-angle optics have a total visual field of 90° (this field is angled 30° with respect to the optical axis). Because the viewing angle is relatively small and the visual field is 90°, a 30° arthroscope still views principally along the optical axis, and so the surgeon sees the structure toward which the scope is advanced.

A 70° arthroscope also has a total visual field of 90°, but the very oblique viewing angle does not permit visualization along the optical axis. As a result, the surgeon cannot see the structures that lie in the path of the advancing scope directly **(Fig. 3)**.

Barrel Length

Arthroscopes are available in various barrel lengths, depending on the manufacturer. A barrel length of 18 cm is recommended for knee arthroscopy.

Diameter

The diameter of the arthroscope is determined by the dimensions of the lens system, the fiberoptics, and the metal barrel. Arthroscopes are available in various

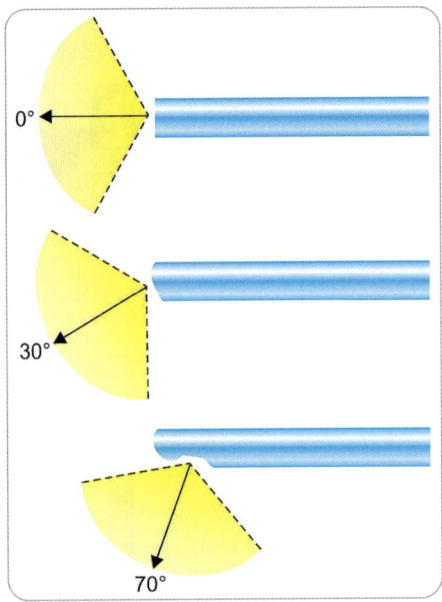

FIG. 3: Viewing angles of different scopes.

diameters. Standard arthroscopes have diameters ranging from 1.7 to 4 mm. The 4-mm arthroscope is standardly used for knee arthroscopy.

Image Quality

Image quality is an important criterion that, unfortunately, is frequently neglected and is difficult to evaluate. The image transmitted by the scope should have sharp edges (if the camera is properly focused) and adequate brightness. The scope should have satisfactory resolution, i.e., it should be able to discriminate fine surface details. One criterion that is easy to analyze is uniform image brightness. This means that when the arthroscope is used on a bright convex surface, all structures should appear uniformly illuminated from the center of the field to the periphery.

Sterilizability

At one time, arthroscopes had to be sterilized by gas. Today this method is no longer used due to environmental concerns, and arthroscopes are sterilized in steam autoclaves (at 134°C under pressure). Scopes cannot be adequately sterilized with a disinfectant solution. The standard instrument recommended for knee arthroscopy is the 30° wide-angle arthroscope.

■ SHEATH

The sheath, with an inserted blunt obturator, is introduced into the joint in preparation for arthroscopy. Once the sheath has entered the joint, the obturator is replaced by the arthroscope.

Components

The sheath consists of coupler (for securing the obturator or scope), spigot plane (for connecting the inflow and outflow tubing), sheath barrel with suction openings, and an inflow channel for the distention medium **(Fig. 4)**.

A sheath system should satisfy various requirements: Secure and rapid fixation in the coupler, rotating spigot plane, adequate diameter, stationary sheath during scope rotation, smooth transition from obturator to sheath, and smooth transition from scope to sheath.

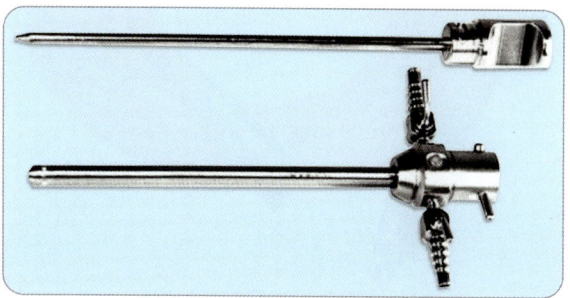

FIG. 4: Sheath and obturator.

◼ ILLUMINATION

To illuminate the joint interior, light from a light source is transmitted into the joint through a light cable and through glass fibers that are integrated into the arthroscope. Either a cold light source or xenon source may be used.

Cold Light Source

These light sources are available in various intensities, with 150 W representing the minimum output necessary for adequate illumination.

Xenon Light Source

Xenon light sources have a higher power output and, with a color temperature of 6000° K, simulating daylight better than a cold light source (color temperature of 4000° K). Xenon light sources should be used in cases where maximum color quality is required, as in the video documentation of arthroscopic findings (digital documentation or video prints). The light source is not switched on until the scope has been inserted into the sheath. Earlier activation of the light source could heat the end of the light cable, scorching the drapes and perhaps burning the patient's leg.

Cables

The light provided by the light source is transmitted to the arthroscope through a light cable (light cord). Either a fiberoptic or fluid type of cable may be used **(Fig. 5)**.

Fiberoptic Cables

These cables transmit light through bundled optical glass fibers and are therefore very flexible. Bending the cable subjects the fibers to varying bending stresses, and constant fiber breakage occurs even during normal use. Significant loss of light transmission does not occur, however, until >50% of the fibers have been

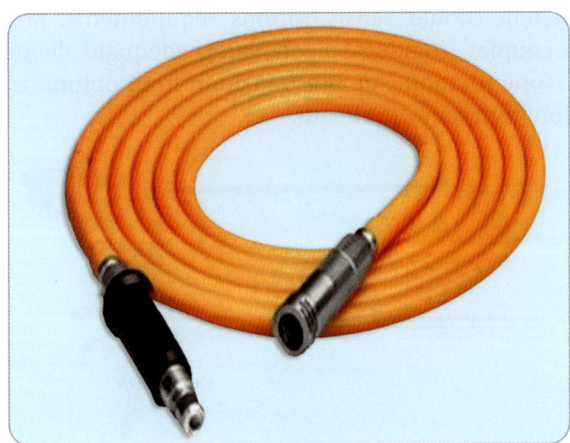

FIG. 5: Light cable.

damaged. Fiberoptic cables are easier to obtain than fluid cables, and they are also easier to sterilize (autoclavable). The cables are available in various lengths. Normally, a length of 150–180 cm is recommended for knee arthroscopy.

Fluid Cables

Fluid cables consist of a plastic tube filled with a special fluid that conducts light 40–50% more efficiently than fiberoptic cables. Fluid cables are less flexible, however, and therefore more difficult to handle. Also, they should be sterilized by immersion in a disinfectant solution rather than autoclaved. Fluid cables transmit light with less intensity loss than fiberoptic cables and give a somewhat bluish touch to the intra-articular structures (the blue wavelengths are transmitted particularly well).

■ VIDEO SYSTEMS

Video Camera

The heart of the video system is the video camera, which consists of the camera itself, the camera cable, and the control unit, which is placed on the arthroscopy cart **(Figs. 6 and 7)**.

Tube Camera

Tube cameras were the first type of cameras developed in the early days of video arthroscopy. These cameras supplied a brilliant image with an exceptional depth of field and excellent color reproduction.

One-chip Camera

This camera is based on the semiconductor chip. Color images are produced by covering the light-sensitive components with appropriate color filters. Image

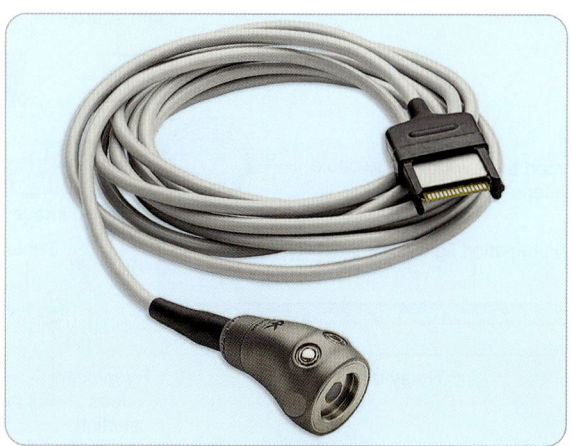

FIG. 6: Camera head.

quality and color reproduction were somewhat poor initially but improved significantly with advances in chip technology, and today these cameras can provide better than 450 lines of resolution.

Three-chip Camera

This camera is equipped with three chips for separately detect and process each of the three primary colors. This arrangement provides an extremely high-quality image with true-to-life color reproduction. The horizontal resolution exceeds 750 lines, so even the finest tissue distinctions can be appreciated. Modern cameras feature digital automatic exposure control, digital color settings, and automatic white balance. They also have a parfocal zoom that controls image focus and size.

An arthroscopic camera should satisfy various requirements: Ergonomic design, mechanism for coupling the camera to the scope, zoom lens, adjustable sharpness, built-in control functions, control unit, camera cable, and sterilization **(Figs. 8 and 9)**.

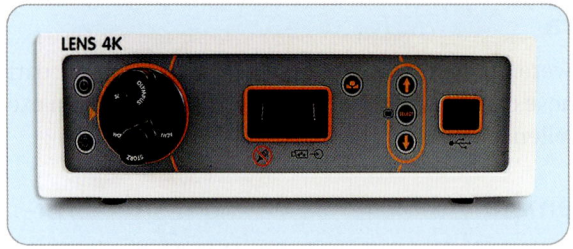

FIG. 7: Camera console.

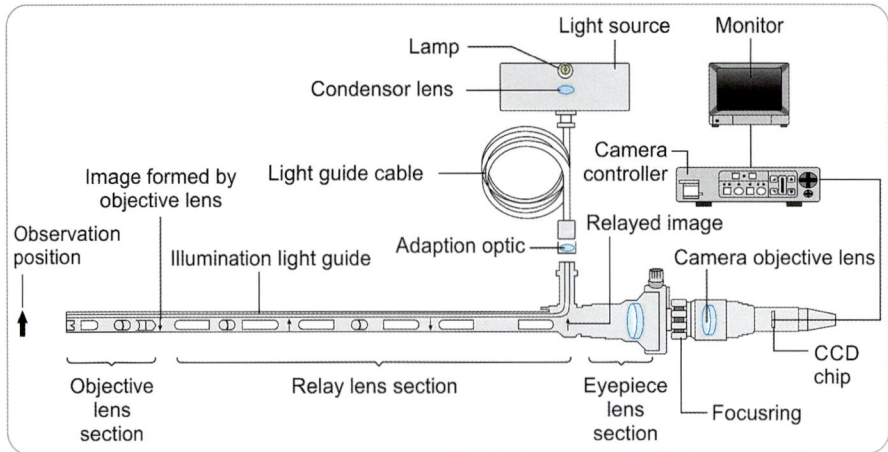

FIG. 8: Components in visualization system.

CHAPTER 1: Introduction to Arthroscopy

■ SHAVER

A motorized instruments set is comprised of control unit, connecting cable between the handpiece and control unit, handpiece **(Fig. 10)**, blades, suction, foot switch **(Fig. 11)**. The shaver handpiece has dual slots for attachment of a shaver blade, may or may not have buttons for hand control, a switch to turn the suction on and off and an outflow port where the suction may be attached **(Fig. 12)**.

Blades

The shaver blade consists of an outer sheath with an open slot at its end and inner blade with serrated edges. The suction attached to the handpiece pulls the tissue into the open slot at the end of the outer sheath. As the inner blade rotates,

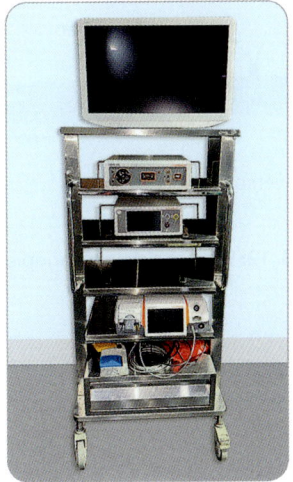

FIG. 9: Arthroscopy trolley.

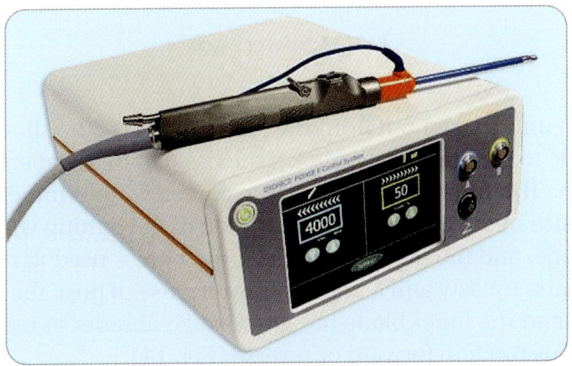

FIG. 10: Shaver console handpiece.

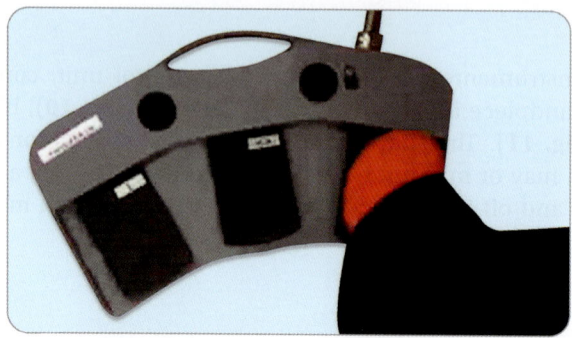

FIG. 11: Shaver foot switch.

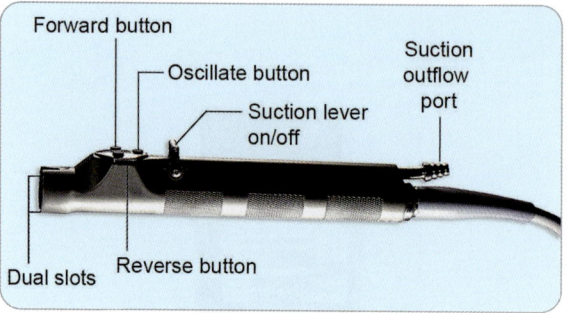

FIG. 12: Parts of a shaver handpiece.

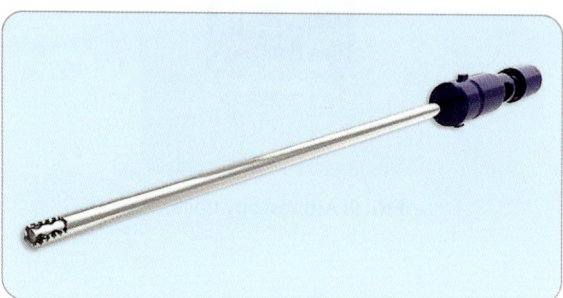

FIG. 13: Shaver blade.

the tissue is cut and sucked out from the joint **(Fig. 13)**. The shaver is run in an oscillating mode to facilitate suctioning of the tissue into the open slot at the end of outer sheath. The function of the shaver blades is determined by operating speed (RPM), size of the cutting window, shape of the cutting window, shape of the rotating blade, and the frequency of use. The burr is used to remove bone as in while doing notchplasty and acromioplasty. In case of burr, the outer sheath is opened at end and the inner blade has got a rough abrader at its tip. The burr is run in continuous rotation forward or reverse **(Fig. 14)**.

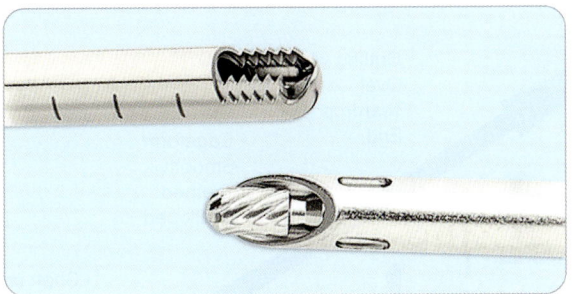

FIG. 14: Shaver blade and burr.

Synovial Resector

This is the most commonly used blade for resecting synovial tissue. The window is oval, and the inner blade is smooth. Even large cartilage fibrillations can be removed, but great care must be taken to preserve normal cartilage areas. Modified forms have a serrated blade and/or a serrated cutting window to produce a more vigorous cutting action.

Meniscus Cutter

The outer tube of this blade is not rounded at the end as in the synovial resector, but has a rectangular window and an angled tip that produces both a side- and end-cutting action. The meniscus cutter is the attachment that is most commonly used for resecting meniscal tissue.

Abrader

This consists of a spherical burr enclosed in an outer tube with a large oval window. It is used to remove osteophytes and other bony structures, smoothing the inlet of bone tunnels, and performing notchplasties.

The various types of shaver blades are shown in **Figure 15**.

■ INDICATIONS

Drive Unit with Blades

Resection of meniscal tissue (meniscus cutter and synovial resector), resection of synovial tissue (synovial resector), resection of scar tissue (meniscus cutter and synovial resector), retrieval of loose bodies (synovial resector), retrieval of small meniscal particles, e.g., following a basket punch resection of meniscal tissue (synovial resector), articular cartilage debridement (note that motorized instruments cannot be controlled as precisely as, electrosurgical instruments or lasers, and therefore risking injury of intact cartilage areas), abrasion of exposed bone to induce fibrocartilage formation (abrader), notchplasty (abrader), removal of osteophytes (abrader), and smoothing of bone tunnel inlets (abrader).

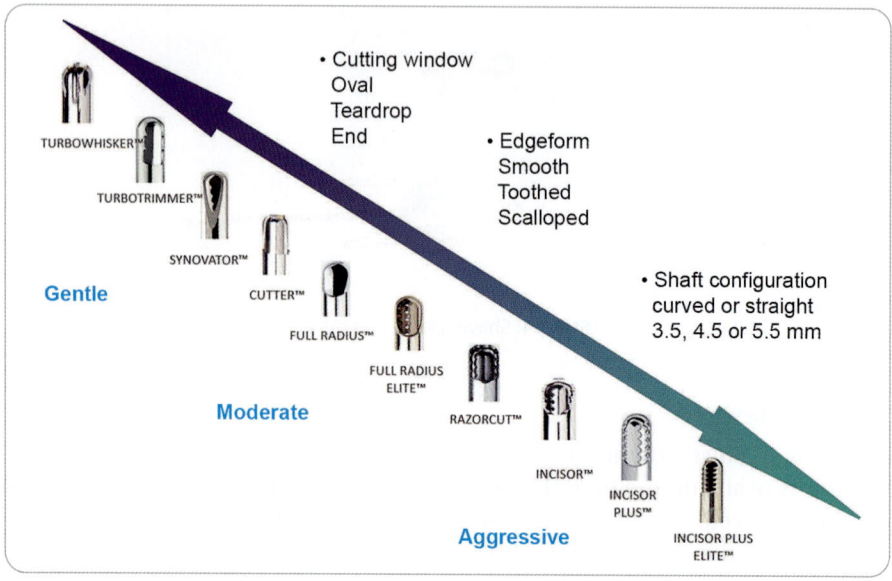

FIG. 15: Types of shaver blade.

Drive Unit with Saw Attachment

Removal of bone blocks from the patella and tibial tuberosity for cruciate ligament reconstruction: bone-tendon-bone (BTB) technique, windowing the bone (e.g., for arthroscopically assisted realignment of upper tibial fractures), and osteotomy (e.g., as part of a corrective or shortening osteotomy).

Drive Unit with Drill Attachment

Drilling bone tunnels [for anterior cruciate ligament (ACL) or posterior cruciate ligament (PCL) reconstruction], harvesting cancellous bone with a hollow burr for cancellous bone grafting (e.g., in osteochondritis dissecans), Kirschner wire insertion (e.g., for temporary fixation of osteochondral fragments), fibrocartilage induction (pridie drilling), drilling holes for bone screws (fixation of ligament substitutes, augmentation materials, repair sutures, and internal fixation devices).

■ SUGGESTED READING

1. Strobel MJ (Ed). Manual of Arthroscopic Surgery. Berlin: Springer; 2002. pp. 4-52.

CHAPTER 2

Knee Positioning, Draping, and Portals

Aditya R Gunjotikar, Vaibhav J Koli, Sachin Yashwant Kale, Prakash D Samant

■ POSITIONING

Ideal positioning should fulfil:
- Accessibility of all joint compartments
- Convenience
- Option for converting to open surgery
- Simple positioning devices
- Free tourniquet access

Essentials for correct positioning:
- Leg holder
- Tourniquet
- Side post
- Foot rest
- Lithotomy stirrup

Straight-leg Position

The straight-leg position **(Figs. 1 and 2)** for arthroscopic surgery meets all the requirements for a simple, fast, and secure positioning technique. A simple side post is mounted on the operating table on the lateral side of the thigh. The side post is positioned about a bandwidth proximal to the base of the patella.

Flexed-knee Position

In this position, the knee is flexed 90° in a padded leg holder. This provides a medial fulcrum so that both varus and valgus stresses can be applied to the knee joint. This positioning technique is disadvantageous in that extra equipment is needed (leg holder) **(Figs. 3 to 6)**.

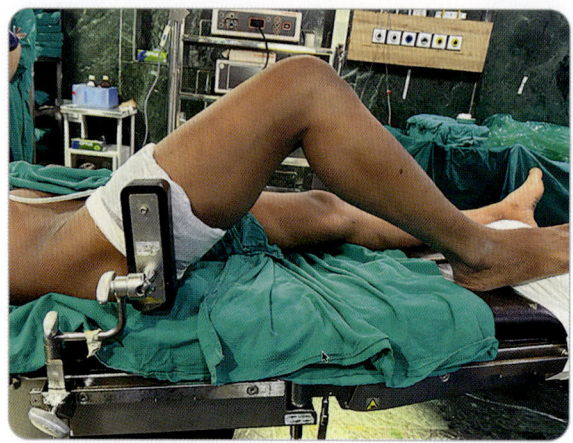

FIG. 1: Supine knee position (flexion).

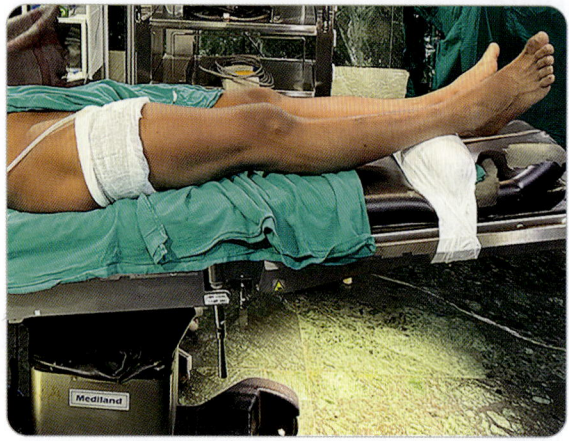

FIG. 2: Supine knee position (extension).

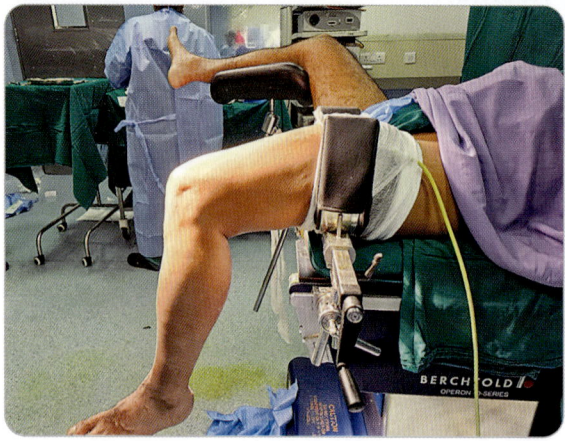

FIG. 3: Leg-hanging knee position (flexion).

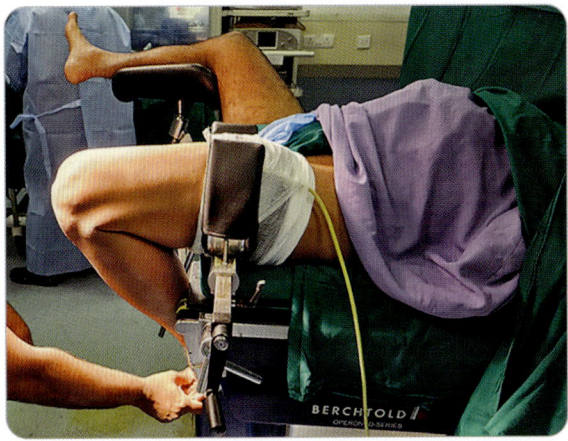

FIG. 4: Leg-hanging knee position (hyperflexion).

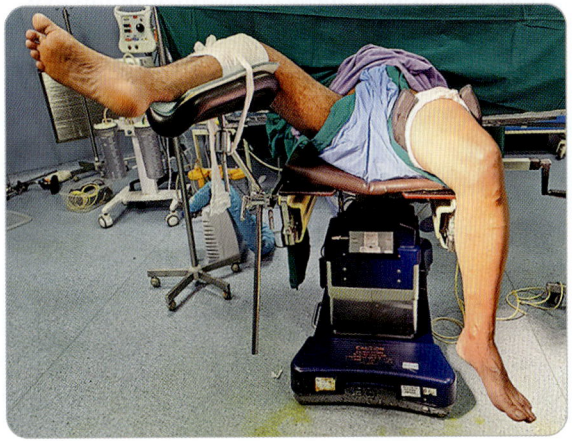

FIG. 5: Well-padded and placed contralateral leg.

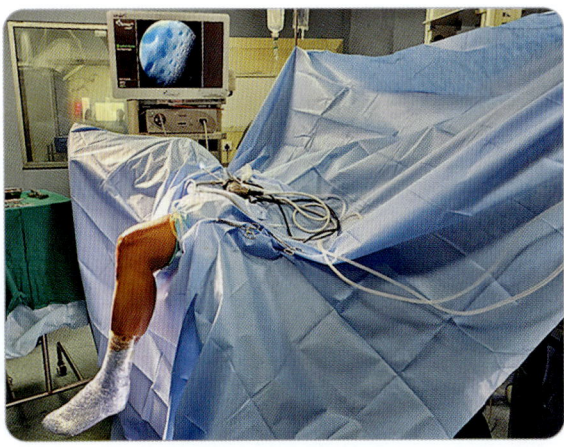

FIG. 6: Post final draping.

Tourniquet Placement

The pneumatic tourniquet is placed on the proximal third of the thigh or at the junction of the proximal and middle thirds. The shorter and thicker the thigh, the more proximal the tourniquet should be placed, especially if an anterior cruciate ligament (ACL) reconstruction is planned. After the tourniquet has been applied, its distal end is covered with a waterproof adhesive drape to keep irrigating fluid and antiseptic solution from getting between the tourniquet and leg **(Figs. 7A and B)**.

■ DRAPING

Since arthroscopy is performed in a fluid-distended joint, the entire surgical field must be covered with waterproof drapes. Water-resistant disposable materials are available for this purpose. Since both the surgical field and the instrument table require waterproof draping, it is convenient to use disposable drape packs that include various sterile drapes in addition to waterproof gowns **(Figs. 8A and B)**.

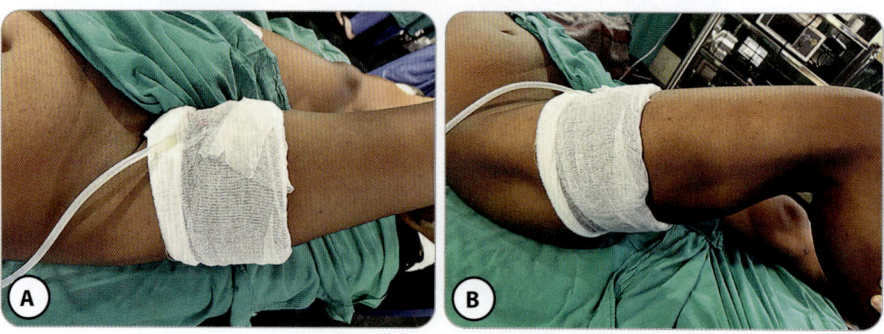

FIGS. 7A AND B: Tourniquet placement.

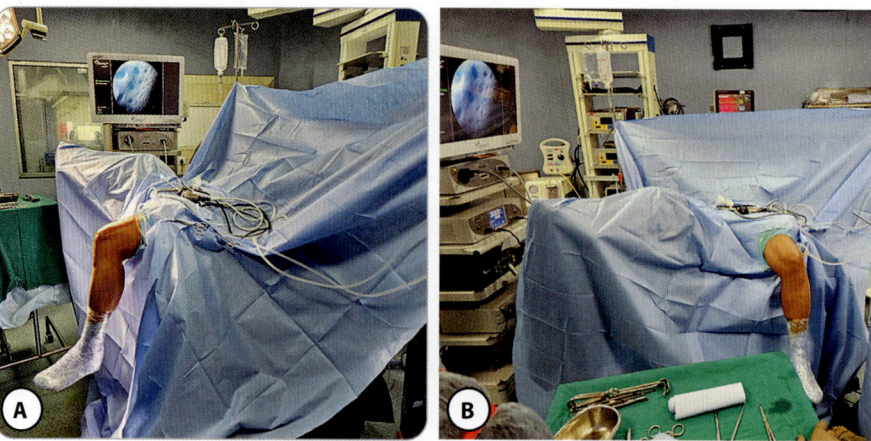

FIGS. 8A AND B: Post final draping.

Draping for Arthroscopic Surgery

The skin is prepared from the level of the tourniquet down to and including the foot. The leg is elevated, and a standard surgical drape is placed under the leg and secured at the front of the thigh with a towel clamp. The prepped leg is then lowered, and the entire surgical fields covered with a waterproof extremity sheet. This sheet has a rubber-lined aperture through which the foot, lower leg, knee joint, and distal thigh are passed. The foot is covered with a waterproof adhesive drape or shod with a rubber glove **(Figs. 9 and 10)**.

Draping for Cruciate Ligament Reconstructions (ACL and PCL)

After the tourniquet is applied, the leg is sterile prepared, and sterile drapes are placed around the leg from below and from above and secured at the level of the thigh. Next the leg is draped with an extremity sheet as described above. The

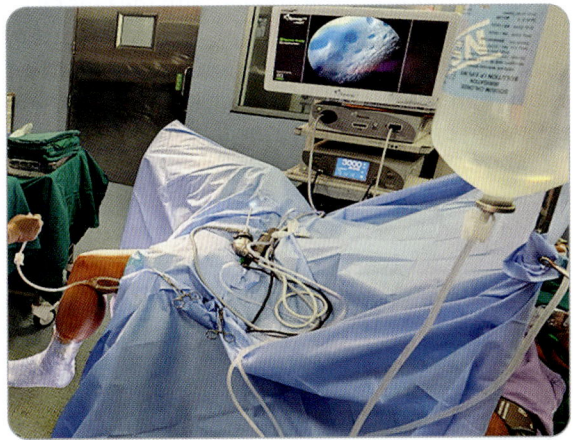

FIG. 9: Set-up.

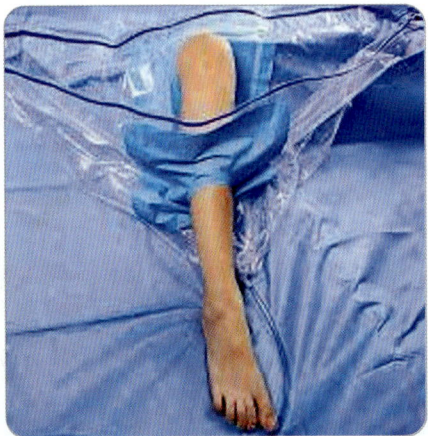

FIG. 10: Bag set-up.

lower leg is then covered with a waterproof disposable towel, which is secured by wrapping a bandage around it. Since cruciate ligament operations require manipulations of the lower leg, elaborate draping of the lower leg is necessary to ensure that the drapes will not slide down at an inopportune time.

Draping the Video Camera

Because video cameras are not autoclavable and should not be immersed in liquid, they are enclosed in a sterile, disposable plastic sleeve to permit sterile handling **(Figs. 11A and B)**.

Draping Steps

Surgical draping for knee arthroscopy is performed in layers. With an assistant holding the leg, the first layer is applied by affixing a sticky drape first with the tails going up, placed just distal to the plastic drape applied before preparation of the leg. Next, a second sticky drape may be applied with the tails facing down, angled so the drape covers the ipsilateral arm board. Finally, an arthroscopy drape is positioned over the foot. This generally has a hole or diaphragm that seals the arthroscopic fluid and prevents it from leaking up under the tourniquet or off the arthroscopic field. As an option, an impermeable stockinette may be placed over the foot to seal it off from the arthroscopic field. The stockinette may be held in position with a Coban wrap or an elastic bandage. The leg is then lowered to the bed, and, at this point, the surgeon or assistant will elevate the post.

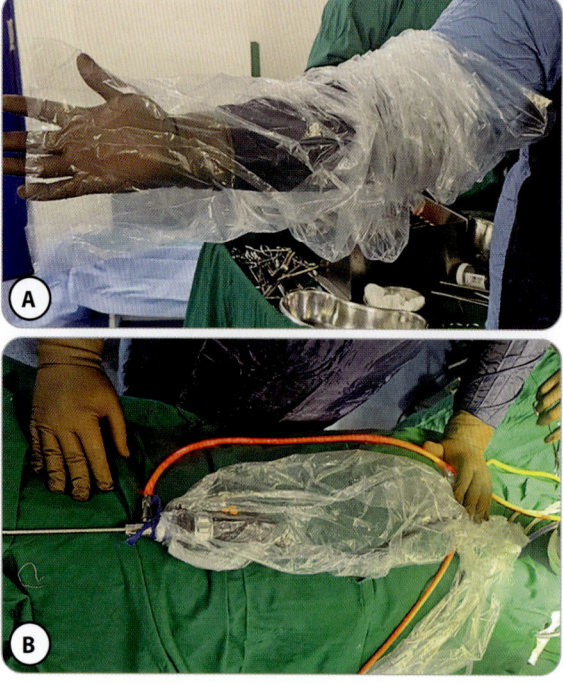

FIGS. 11A AND B: Camera cover.

PORTALS

Technique for Creating Portals

Position

The knee joint is flexed approximately 70°, and the foot or lower leg is placed stable to maintain constant flexion angle.

Identification of Anatomic Structures (Fig. 12)

First, the patellar apex, patellar tendon, and lateral femoral condyle are identified by palpation. The lateral border of the patellar tendon, the medial circumference of the lateral femoral condyle, and distally by the superior rim of the anterior horn of the lateral meniscus, which is palpated, form the lateral triangle. The patellar apex provides a key landmark for placement of the arthroscope portal.

Portal Site

The optimum site for the arthroscope portal is determined by reference to the palpable anatomic structures and any anatomic peculiarities that are present. The high anterolateral portal is considered the standard viewing portal in arthroscopic knee surgery.

Infiltration with Local Anesthetic

Once the optimum site for the arthroscope portal has been selected, it is infiltrated with a local anesthetic (bupivacaine 0.25%) containing 1:200,000 epinephrine. Approximately 5 mL of solution is sufficient.

Skin Incision

A vertical skin incision approximately 5 mm long is made with a scalpel (No. 11 blade).

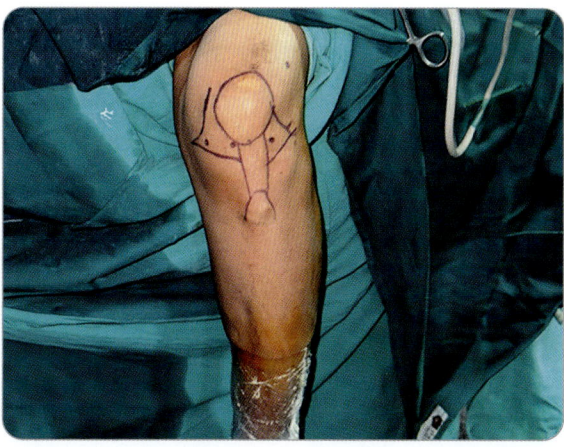

FIG. 12: Skin markings.

Insertion of the Sheath (Fig. 13)

The arthroscope sheath armed with a blunt obturator is introduced into the joint. The sheath is inserted with a careful rotary motion, initially directing the sheath toward the notch.

Extension of the Knee Joint

When the sheath and blunt obturator have penetrated the fibrous capsule and tissue resistance declines, the knee joint is extended and the sheath is carefully advanced into the medial portion of the superior recess.

First, suction the fluid collection from the joint. If infection is suspected, send the aspirate or smear for bacteriologic and histologic analysis. Whether the effusion is serous or bloody, it should be removed as completely as possible. Large blood clots may clog the irrigation opening in the sheath. Before the suction is turned on, remove the blunt obturator and manually occlude the sheath opening. Hemarthrosis can be flushed from the joint by alternating inflow and outflow of the irrigating fluid. This is supported by manually manipulating ("milking") the superior recess and posterior recess from the outside to mobilize the clots and facilitate their removal.

Types of Portals

High Anterolateral Portal (Fig. 14)

This portal is placed adjacent to the lateral border of the patellar tendon at the level of the patellar apex. This is the usual viewing portal in knee arthroscopy.

Anteromedial Portal (Fig. 15)

This portal is placed at the level of the patellar apex medial to the patellar tendon (half patella tendon's breadth away, in line with the AL portal). This is the usual instrument portal. A spinal needle is first inserted at the site of skin incision. The

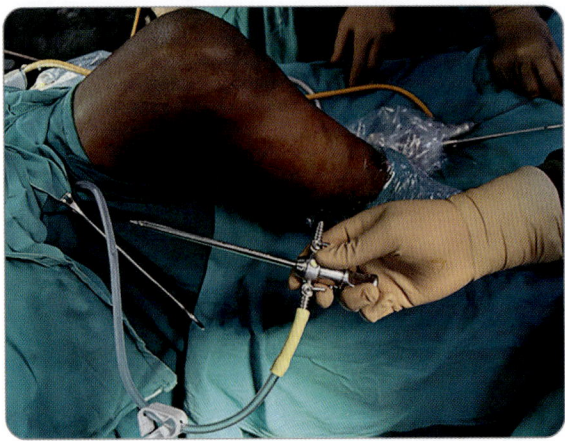

FIG. 13: Sheath set up.

CHAPTER 2: Knee Positioning, Draping, and Portals

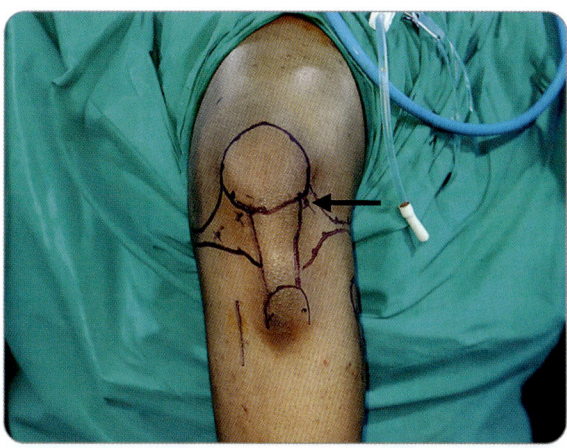

FIG. 14: Anterolateral portal (black arrow).

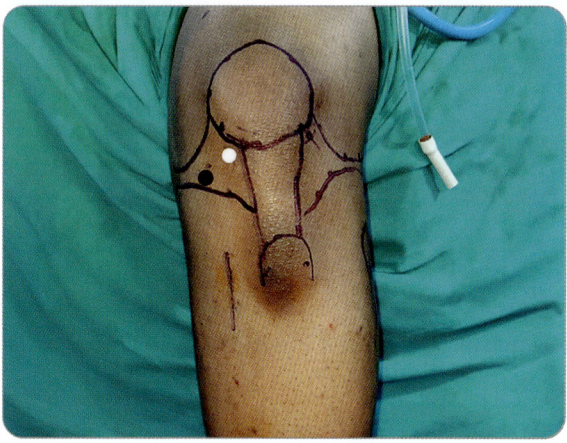

FIG. 15: Anteromedial portal (white circle) and accessory anteromedial portal (black circle).

tip of the of the needle is visualized and if the trajectory of the needle is satisfactory then the portal is taken with a knife.

At times, a proper trajectory to drill the femoral tunnel may not be achieved through a standard anteromedial portal. In this situation, an accessory anteromedial portal may be taken to drill the femoral tunnel. The accessory anteromedial portal is more medial and lower than the standard anteromedial portal. A corresponding accessory anterolateral portal may be taken in line with the accessory anteromedial portal.

Medial Suprapatellar Portal (Fig. 16)

This portal is placed slightly proximal to the superior border of the patella. The danger of this approach is the potential for injury of the vastus medialis muscle, especially its distal portion (vastus medialis obliquus).

Lateral Suprapatellar Portal (Fig. 16)

A lateral suprapatellar portal placed just above the superior border of the patella is necessary when performing a complete synovectomy.

Posteromedial Portal (Fig. 17)

This portal is placed with the knee flexed 90°, and adequate joint distention is required. The first, essential step is to inspect the posteromedial capsule. This is done by passing the arthroscope posteromedially through the intercondylar area with the knee in slight flexion. From this vantage point the posterior cruciate ligament (PCL) forms the lateral boundary of the field while the medial aspect of the medial femoral condyle forms the medial

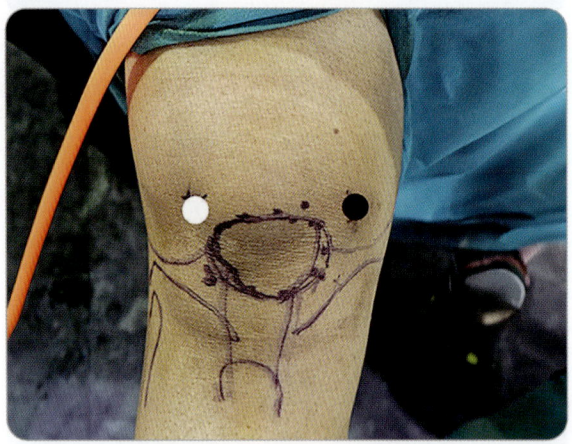

FIG. 16: Medial (black circle) and lateral suprapatellar portal (white circle) with knee in extension.

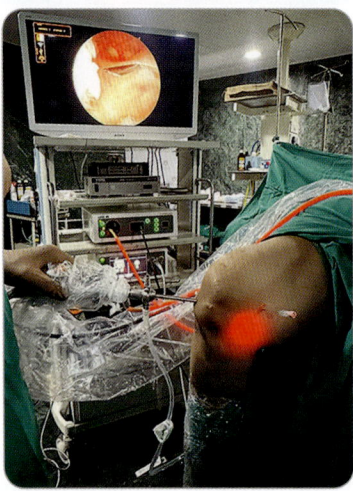

FIG. 17: Needle technique for posteromedial (PM) portal.

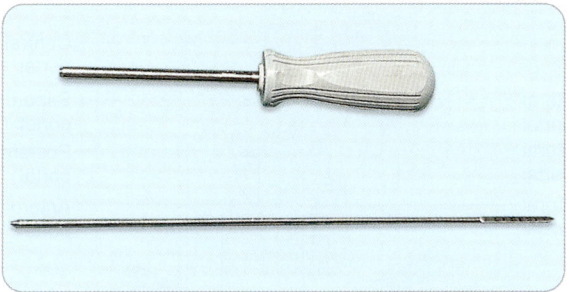

FIG. 18: Switching stick and dilator.

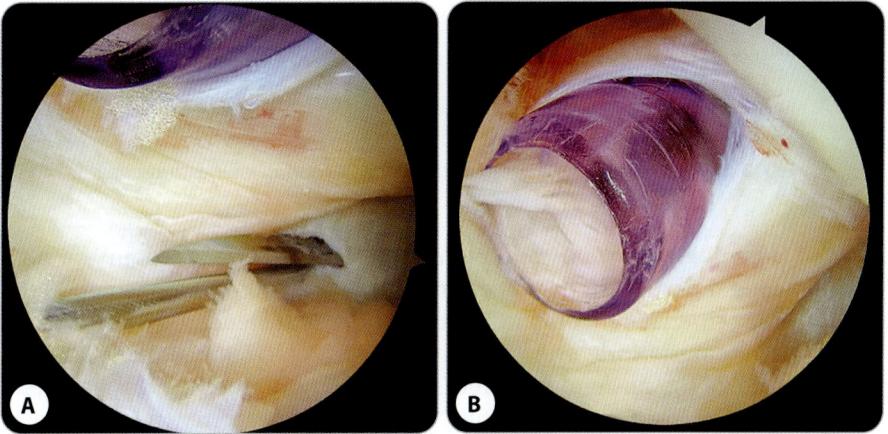

FIGS. 19A AND B: Inside view.

boundary. Once the arthroscope is passed in the posteromedial area, we could be able to visualize the transillumination **(Figs. 17 to 19)**, which helps us to locate the posteromedial recess. The point of needle insertion is identified by external digital palpation, and a needle is inserted into the recess to confirm that all essential structures can be reached from the posteromedial portal. This portal is placed approximately 1–2 fingers width proximal to the joint space.

Posterolateral Portal (Fig. 20)

The creation of a posterolateral portal begins with arthroscopic inspection of the posterolateral recess. One of two viewing portals may be used:
1. *Medial arthroscope portal*: The arthroscope is first introduced through a "standard" high anterolateral portal. Then a switching rod is inserted through a high medial portal, and the knee is moved to the figure-four position while the switching rod is passed in front of the ACL into the posterolateral recess. Next, the arthroscope is removed from the anterolateral portal, and the sheath is advanced over the switching rod into the posterolateral recess, which is then inspected.

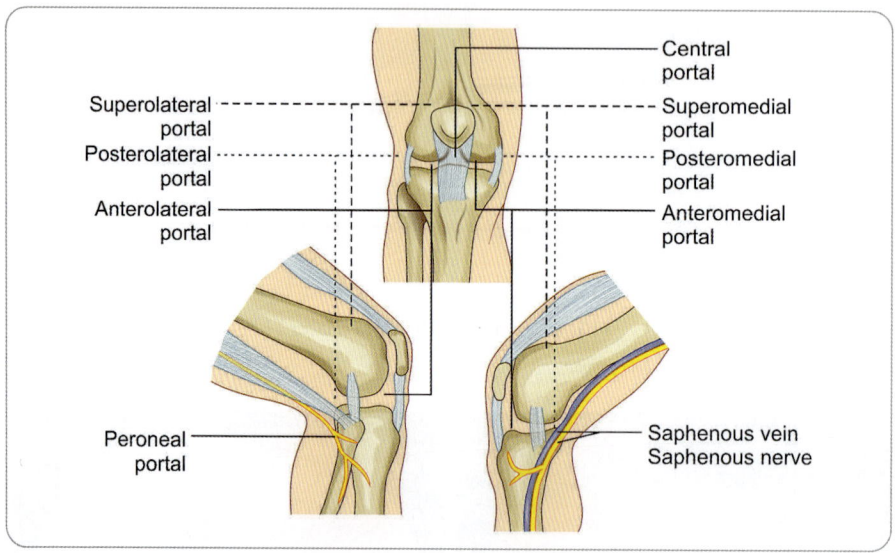

FIG. 20: Illustration of few commonly taken portals during knee arthroscopy.

2. *High anterolateral arthroscope portal*: The arthroscope is left in the high anterolateral portal and the knee is moved to the figure-four position. If the joint is lax, the lateral compartment will be well distended. By passing the arthroscope posteriorly over the posterior horn of the lateral meniscus, one can visualize the posterolateral recess. A large portion of the posterolateral recess can be inspected by rotating the scope, but the view may not be as complete as when the scope is inserted through a high medial instrument portal.

The extent of the posterolateral capsule is determined by palpation, and a needle is inserted. The needle should always be inserted proximal to the biceps femoris muscle to preserve the peroneal nerve. After the skin is incised, the subcutaneous tissue and capsule are spread open with a small forceps, and the operating instrument is inserted.

■ SUGGESTED READINGS

1. Strobel MJ. Manual of arthroscopic surgery. Berlin: Springer; 2002. pp. 52-72.
2. Ward BD, Lubowitz JH. Basic knee arthroscopy part 1: patient positioning. Arthrosc Tech. 2013;2(4):e497-9.
3. Ward BD, Lubowitz JH. Basic knee arthroscopy part 2: surface anatomy and portal placement. Arthrosc Tech. 2013;2(4):e501-2.

CHAPTER 3

Grafts

*Sandeep Narayan Deore, Rohit Mahesh Sane,
Shikhar D Singh, Sanjay B Dhar, Sachin Yashwant Kale*

■ INTRODUCTION

Several graft options are available—patellar tendon (the central one-third with attached bone plugs), semitendinosus tendon (ST tendon), ST and gracilis tendons, quadriceps tendon, and peroneus longus tendon (PL tendon).

Graft remodeling is time-consuming but well researched. The success of an anterior cruciate ligament (ACL) reconstruction depends critically on the biological remodeling of the graft, which basically can be described as a "free-grafted avascular connective tissue structure." Initially, the graft becomes partially necrotic before undergoing a remodeling process that resembles the stages of wound healing. It is reasonable to assume, therefore, that a graft in the human knee significantly alters its mechanical properties and histologic structure within a short period of time. It remains unclear whether this tissue structure becomes increasingly "ligamentous" and approaches the normal histologic structure of the ACL.

Patellar Tendon (Bone-tendon-bone)

One of the most widely used graft for ACL reconstruction is the central one-third of the patellar tendon **(Fig. 1)**. This graft includes bone plugs from the patella

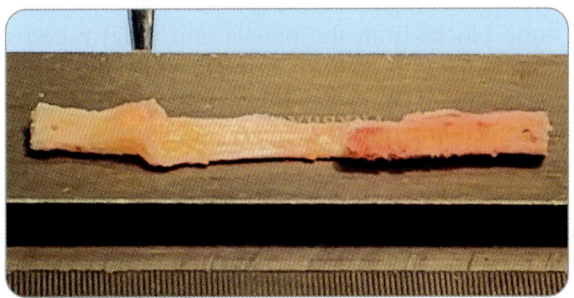

FIG. 1: Bone-patellar tendon-bone graft.

and tibial tuberosity to provide a very stable primary fixation that allows for early motion and weight bearing (modulus of elasticity—225 MPa).

Surgical Technique

Anterior paramedial incision is taken between patella and tibial tuberosity. Subcutaneous plane is created for rotating window. Patellar tendon is identified.

Paratenon is incised in the midline to expose the tendon. Central third of patellar tendon along with patellar and tibial bone plug is marked with skin marker. Central third patellar tendon is incised full thickness extending to bony attachments. Patellar bone plug (size 10 mm by 7 mm) is harvested with help of 5-mm saw blade to the depth of 7 mm in triangular fashion to avoid patellar fracture. After dissecting central patellar tendon, tibial bone plug (size 20 by 10 mm) is harvested with 5-mm saw blade. In each bone plug, two drill holes are made for passage of ultra braid or fiber wires. Average length of the harvested graft varies between 70 and 90 mm. The extra bone removed from the bone plugs is filled in the donor site and remaining tendon is sutured tightly to avoid fluid extravasation.

Advantages

- Variable graft width. Normally a sufficiently wide patellar tendon is available for graft harvest. The usual graft width is 8–10 mm.
- *Availability*: The patellar tendon is always available and shows little anatomic variation. This permits a constant and technically simple harvesting technique.
- *Bone to bone healing and strong primary fixation*: The bone plugs allow for strong primary fixation of the graft. This method provides high primary stability.
- *Preservation of active internal rotation*: Because the tendons responsible for internal rotation of the knee are not violated, harvesting the graft does not compromise internal rotation.
- *Weakening the antagonist*: The quadriceps femoris muscle is the strongest antagonist of the ACL, and so weakening of the muscle during the graft healing period is considered beneficial.

Disadvantages

Donor site morbidity includes several problem areas:
- *Bony defects*: Because a longitudinal strip is harvested from the patellar tendon along with bone blocks from the patella and tibial tuberosity, a palpable bone defect and fat pad herniation during knee flexion can be felt in skinny patients giving cosmetic concerns. This can be avoided by cancellous bone grafting in the defects and proper repair of paratenon.
- *Compromise of the extensor apparatus*: A quadriceps deficit of approximately 15% persists for up to 1 year. This is particularly disabling to athletes who rely on an intact extensor apparatus (skiers, basketball players, and volleyball players). A well-structured supervised physiotherapy is required to strengthen extensor mechanism.

- *Anterior knee pain*: There are multiple reasons for anterior knee pain—retropatellar crepitus in patients with preexisting patellofemoral cartilage disease, scarring of the infrapatellar fat pad, scar tissue in the donor defect, and patellar apex syndrome. This may lead to difficulty in kneeling down. This can be prevented by timely mobilization on the knee and local physical therapy to prevent scar formation. Scarring of skin to underlying tibial tuberosity and patellar apex can lead to limitation of knee flexion. This can be prevented by taking paramedian or oblique skin incision.
- *Risk of patellar fracture*: A longitudinal or transverse fracture of the patella may occur when the patellar bone block is harvested. If a large bone block is removed, the patella may be fractured weeks or months later by a trivial trauma.
- *Injury to the pes anserinus*: If the bone-tendon-bone (BTB) graft is long, the bone plug must either be placed high in the femoral tunnel or, if the femoral end of the graft is fixed with an interference screw on the articular side, the tibial tunnel must be started at a very low level. This may cause injury to the pes anserinus complex. If a revision is necessary, the ST tendon may be unsuitable for use or very difficult to dissect and harvest.
- *Risk of cyclops syndrome*: The volume of the graft increases during remodeling, and scar tissue forming anterior to the distal attachment site can create a mechanical block to extension (cyclops syndrome).

Contraindications to the Bone-tendon-bone Technique

These are previous surgery on the patellar tendon, Osgood–Schlatter disease, patella baja, significant patellofemoral osteoarthritis, and prior ACL reconstruction of the opposite knee using the BTB technique.

Hamstrings: Semitendinosus and Gracilis Tendon

Semitendinosus is one other commonly used graft.

Given the disadvantages of the BTB technique listed above, the ST tendon is becoming increasingly popular as an alternative graft material for ACL reconstruction.

Advantages

- *Small incision*: The ST tendon can be harvested through an incision only about 3 cm long.
- *No compromise of the extensor apparatus*: The quadriceps muscle, patellar tendon, and tibial tuberosity remain intact.
- No incidence of anterior knee pain as found in BTB
- *Favorable elastic modulus*: The three- or four-strand ST tendon graft has an elastic modulus similar to that of the normal ACL (modulus of elasticity—145 MPa, native—120 MPa).
- *Less risk of cyclops syndrome*: Less scar formation occurs during graft remodeling than in the BTB technique.

Disadvantages
- *Posterior thigh ecchymosis* due to hematoma at the donor site.
- *Weakening of the agonist*: The ST muscle is an important part of the hamstring group, which is the principal agonist of the ACL.
- *Injury to saphenous nerve* leading to hypoesthesia over anterolateral border of the leg. Oblique incision is preferable to avoid this complication.
- Prior surgery around proximal tibia with metallic implants may make it difficult to find the anatomical landmarks for tendon harvesting.
- Premature amputation of the ST due to incomplete release of the fibrous bands. Chubby patients may have smaller tendons.

Surgical Technique

Incision: Three finger width below the joint line and medial to the tibial tuberosity. Anatomy of pes anserinus is such that round-shaped gracilis and flat ST are covered by a curtain of sartorius. Finger can be rolled over round gracilis tendon as an identification landmark **(Figs. 2 and 3)**.

There are two methods to approach the hamstrings. In the first method, horizontal incision is taken between rounded gracilis and flat ST so that either of them can be harvested depending upon the need. In the second method, a reverse "L" incision is taken with horizontal limb at upper border of gracilis and vertical limb cutting the attachments of ST and gracilis so that both tendons are detached from insertion **(Figs. 4 to 6)**.

Care must be taken not to injure medial collateral ligament just beneath the pes anserinus.

Mixter forceps is used to lift up the ST. Ethibond is rolled around the tendon.

The tibial attachment is cut parallel to the fibers to include periosteum. ST is pulled to expose the vincula connecting to the medial gastrocnemius. Care is taken to cut all bands connecting the two structures. Saphenous nerve need to be protected **(Fig. 7)**.

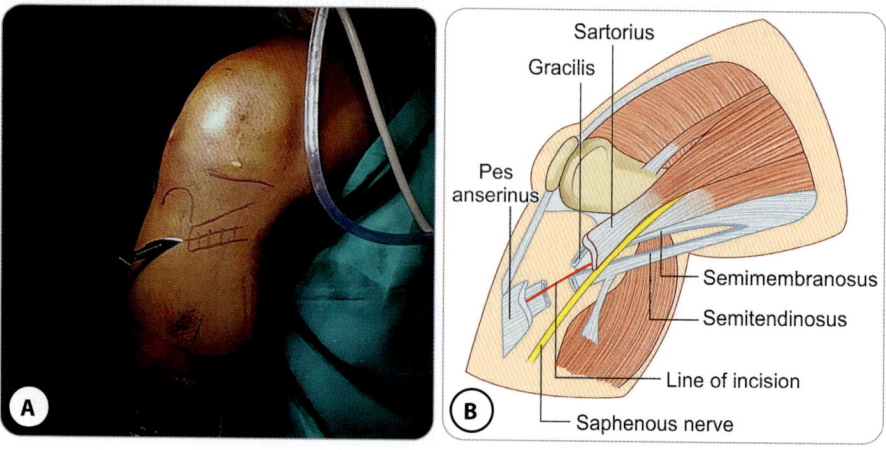

FIGS. 2A AND B: Surface anatomy and skin marking.

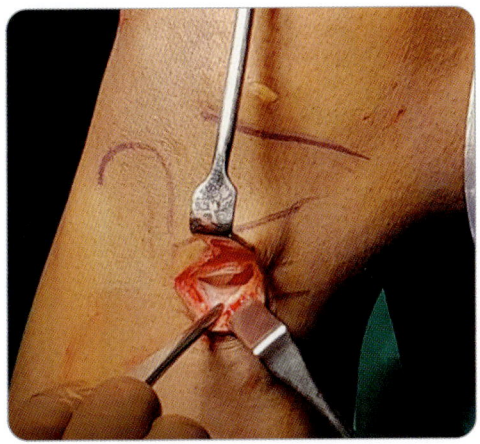

FIG. 3: Split between gracilis and semitendinosus.

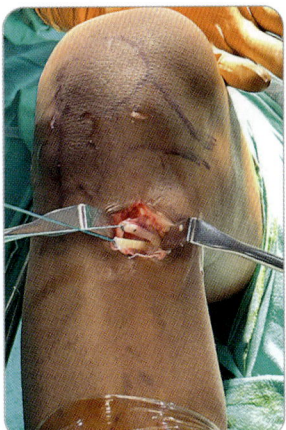

FIG. 4: Isolation of tendinosis and gracilis.

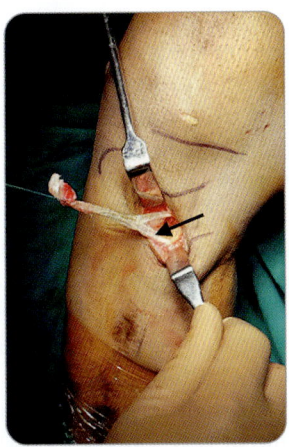

FIG. 5: Isolation of semitendinosus with fibrous band connecting to gastrocnemius.

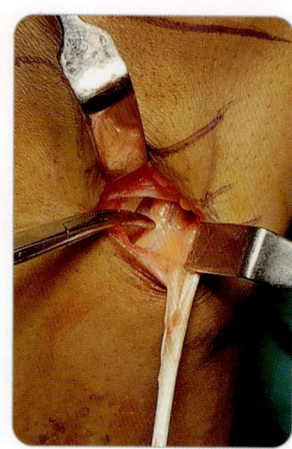

FIG. 6: Medial collateral ligament below pes anserinus to be protected.

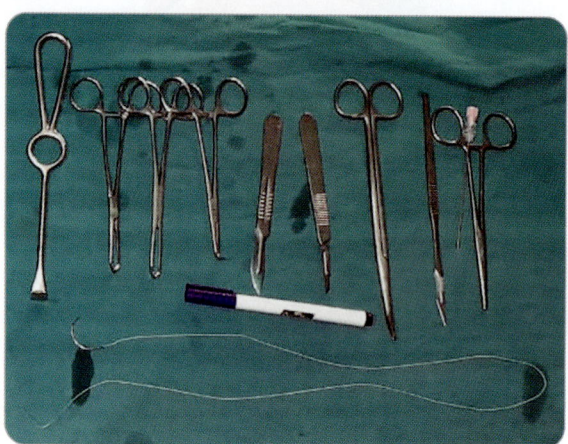

FIG. 7: Instruments required for graft harvesting.

A close-ended tendon stripper is passed around the ST to strip the tendon off the muscle fibers. Average length we obtain is between 270 and 300 mm. Open-ended tendon stripper can be used if tibial attachment is to be kept intact in procedures like medial collateral ligament reconstruction.

Similar procedure is repeated for gracilis tendon. The second method to harvest the tendons is through an "L"-shaped incision starting from the superior border of gracilis to the vertical tibial crest where both the tendons are attached. With the help of blunt periosteum, the muscles fibers are stripped off the tendon. Depending upon the length, the graft is a folded on itself over fiber–wire loop three to four times, the aim being diameter greater than 8 mm. The graft is mounted on the adjustable or fixed loop and button, and kept for pretensioning on the graft board, covered by a vancomycin-soaked sterile gauze piece **(Figs. 8 and 9)**.

If the ST tendon is very thin or very short (< 24 cm), the gracilis tendon can be harvested to make a combined graft.

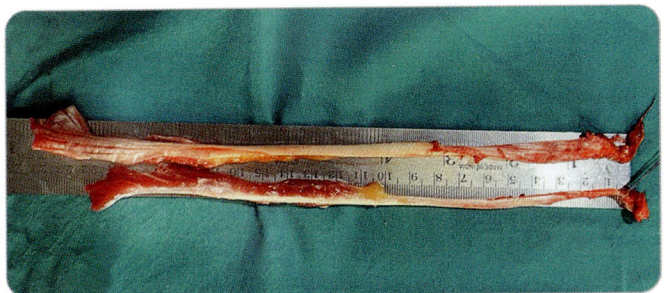

FIG. 8: Harvested tendon graft.

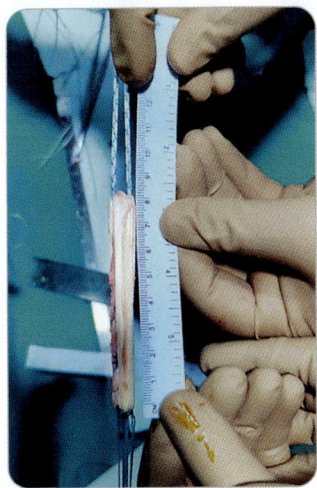

FIG. 9: Measurement of graft length.

Quadriceps Tendon

Increasingly, the quadriceps tendon is being used for ACL and posterior cruciate ligament (PCL) reconstructions.

Surgical Procedure

A 3–4 cm suprapatellar midline vertical incision is taken. Subcutaneous plane is created to make a sliding window to increase work area. Paratenon is incised. Medial and lateral border of quadriceps tendon is identified. Central third tendon is incised at 8 mm depth keeping deep tendon intact. This central strip is extended vertically up to a length of 80 mm and cut. Distal part of the graft involves area up to periosteum over patella. We can also take 10 mm of patellar bone plug with the help of a saw. After harvesting the graft, remnant tendon is sutured together with No. 1 Vicryl in double layer to avoid saline seepage during arthroscopy **(Figs. 10 to 12)**.

Recently, minimally invasive methods of quadriceps harvesting are available which involve a cylindrical calibrated harvester and graft cutter at the end of the tube **(Fig. 13)**.

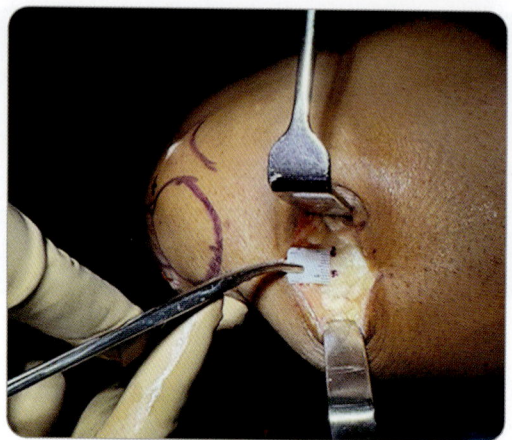

FIG. 10: 10-mm wide graft measured.

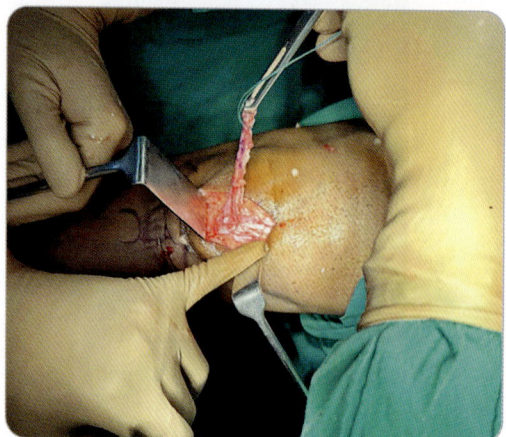

FIG. 11: Central third quadriceps tendon dissected.

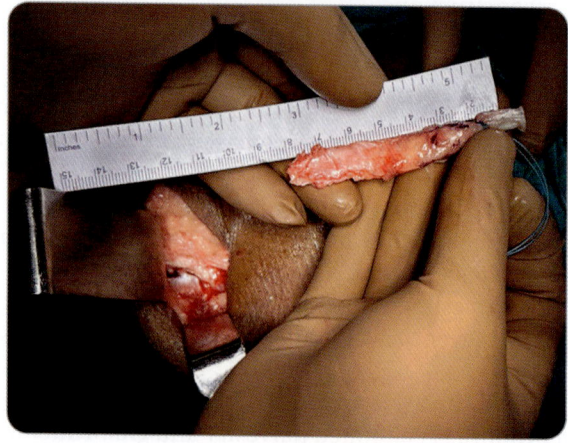

FIG. 12: 75-mm graft harvested.

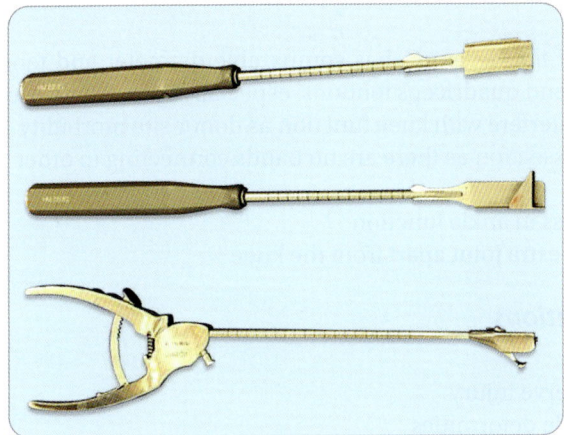

FIG. 13: Quadriceps tendon harvesting instruments.

Advantages
- *Larger cross-section of the graft*: The quadriceps tendon has the same width as the patellar tendon but a larger cross-sectional area with relatively better initial strength, and hence is preferred for procedures like PCL reconstruction.
- *Bony fixation*: The patellar bone block allows for bony fixation of the graft at the level of the joint space (e.g., in the femoral tunnel).
- *Less donor site morbidity*: Use of the quadriceps tendon is associated with less donor site morbidity than the patellar tendon.
- *Less irritation of patellofemoral joint*: Because the quadriceps tendon attaches to the base of the patella over a very broad area, and therefore, the patella is weakened on its broader side when the graft is harvested, there is less impact on the femoropatellar joint then when the central third of the patellar tendon (BTB technique) is used.

Disadvantages
- *Extra incision*: Because of its location, the graft must always be harvested through a separate skin incision.
- Quadriceps wasting and weakness is a potential complication and hence robust physiotherapy protocol is required.
- *Fluid outflow*: As roof of the suprapatellar pouch is opened, watertight repair of the quadriceps defect in two layers is required to prevent fluid outflow.

Peroneus Longus Graft

Peroneus longus is harvested from ankle region. This graft choice is considered as a spare graft for revision surgery and female patients with obesity and short stature.

Advantages
- *Longer and thicker graft*—has comparable diameter and tensile strength to hamstring and quadriceps tendons, especially useful in revision surgeries.
- Does not interfere with knee function as donor site morbidity
- Minimal dissection as there are no bands connecting to other muscles unlike in the knee
- No weakness in ankle function
- Surgery on extra joint apart from the knee

Contraindications
- Flat foot
- Peroneal nerve injury
- Foot or ankle deformities

Surgical Procedure
With foot in international rotation, a 2-cm incision is taken on the lateral part of the ankle just behind the lateral malleolus. After achieving hemostasis, peroneal sheath is incised longitudinally **(Figs. 14 to 16)**. Care is taken to avoid injury to sural nerve which lies posteriorly. More superficial PL tendon is isolated and tagged with Ethibond No. 5. With foot in everted position, tendon is cut distally. The remnant can be sutured to peroneus brevis or left alone. A tendon stripper is passed along the leg vertically with constant pull on the sutures to receive long and thick tendon. Care is taken to avoid injury to peroneal nerve. As per the need, PL tendon can be tripled or quadrupled as graft for ACL or PCL reconstruction **(Figs. 17 and 18)**.

Synthetic Materials
Various polymeric materials have been used for ACL reconstruction (Nylon, Dacron, Teflon, Trevira, and Gore-Tex). These prosthetic ligaments are specially woven and braided, depending on the manufacturer.

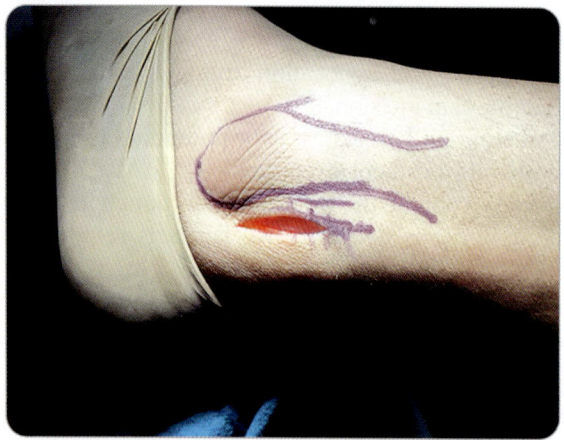

FIG. 14: Incision for peroneus longus tendon taken.

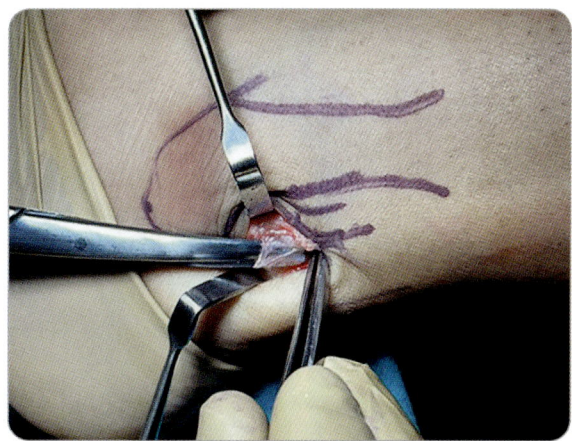

FIG. 15: Peroneus sheath incised longitudinally.

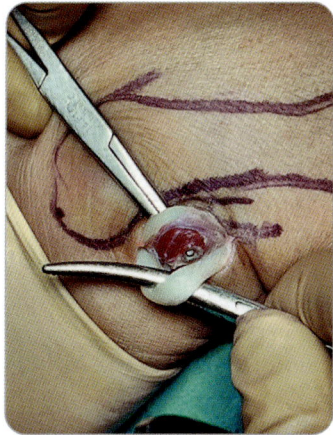

FIG. 16: Peroneus longus and peroneus brevis isolated.

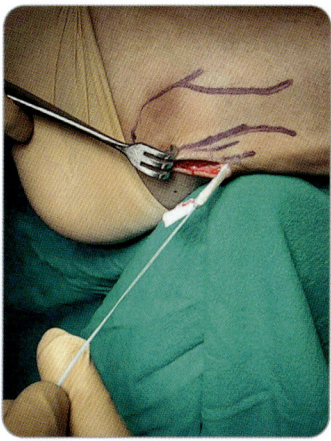

FIG. 17: Harvesting the tendon.

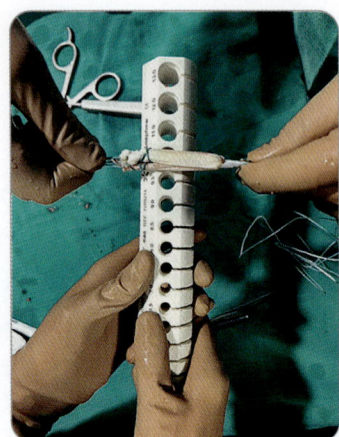

FIG. 18: Measurement of graft diameter.

Disadvantages

- *Poor biocompatibility*: The rupture of a Dacron or Gore-Tex ligament, e.g., incites a characteristic synovitis that causes pain and persistent effusions.
- *Infection*: Relatively higher rate of infection being a foreign material. Complete removal of the synthetic ligament is necessary to relieve the symptoms.
- *High rupture rate*: Approximately, 50% of synthetic ligaments undergo partial or complete rupture within 5 years. Sites of predilection are—the site of emergence from the femoral tunnel, the entry site into the tibial tunnel (bending on flexion and extension), and osteophytes in the intercondylar notch (guillotine like action on extension).
- *High incidence of synovitis*: Some prosthetic ligaments, especially those containing carbon fibers, have very high reported rates of postoperative synovitis.
- *High costs*: The procurement and storage costs can be considerable.
- *Need for a lateral incision*: Because the prosthetic ligaments are not fixed in the bone tunnel with an interference screw, a separate lateral incision is required for the insertion of screws, staples, or both, as recommended by the manufacturer. This extra incision increases the morbidity of the procedure.

Allografts

The use of "cadaveric ligaments" offers a conceivable alternative to prosthetic materials. The main advantage of allografts is the absence of donor site morbidity. An allograft is a useful treatment option, and sometimes the only option, in some revision procedures (e.g., after multiple failed ligament reconstructions) and in patients with multiple injuries (e.g., bilateral ruptures of the ACL and PCL) accompanied by complex peripheral instabilities.

Available options are—tendoachilles and BTB.

TABLE 1: Comparison of different grafts.

Type of graft	Pros	Cons
Autograft		
Bone-patellar tendon-bone (BPTB)	• Strong fixation due to bone plugs • Fast bone-to-bone healing	• Risk of anterior knee pain and kneeling discomfort • Patellar fracture or tendinitis risk
Hamstring tendons	• Minimal donor site morbidity • Smaller incision • High tensile strength	• Slower graft healing • Risk of hamstring weakness • Difficult fixation compared to BPTB
Quadriceps tendon	• Large graft diameter • Lower risk of donor site complications compared to BPTB	• Risk of extensor mechanism weakness • Limited long-term data
Peroneus longus tendon	• Long and strong tendon • Minimal functional deficit after harvest • Easy to harvest	• Limited data on long-term outcomes • Risk of lateral ankle weakness
Allograft:		
Tibialis anterior/posterior or Achilles	• No donor site morbidity • Shorter operative time • Useful for multiligament reconstructions	• Higher risk of graft rejection or infection • Delayed graft incorporation • Expensive
Synthetic grafts	E.g., LARS ligament	• Immediate strength • No donor site morbidity
Xenografts	• Readily available • Avoids donor site morbidity	• Risk of immune rejection • Limited use due to ethical and cultural concerns

(LARS: ligament augmentation and reconstruction system)

Advantages
- No donor site problems
- Always available
- Suitable for revision cases

Disadvantages
- *Immune reaction*: Many recipients have developed chronic synovitis with pain and recurrent effusions.
- *Softened bone at tunnel entrances*: If revision becomes necessary after an allograft reconstruction, marked softening of the bone is typically found at the intra-articular tunnel entrances. This can greatly increase the difficulty of the revision procedure (cancellous bone grafting of the softened areas).

- *Costs*: The procurement and storage costs must be taken into account.
- *Finite risk of HIV/HBV/HCV transmission*: Allograft transmission of human immunodeficiency virus is extremely unlikely, and the risk has been characterized as extremely low in publications. Nevertheless, the risk cannot be completely eliminated.

SUGGESTED READING

1. Strobel MJ. Manual of arthroscopic surgery. Berlin: Springer; 2002. pp. 384-91.

CHAPTER 4

Diagnostic Round (Knee), Indications, and Contraindications

Vaibhav J Koli, Vishal Kumar, Sachin Yashwant Kale, Rohit Mahesh Sane

■ SEQUENCE OF ARTHROSCOPIC EXAMINATION (NO FIXED ORDER)

Superior Recess

The diagnostic arthroscopy starts in the suprapatellar pouch. With the knee in extension, the trochlea is seen in the lower part of the screen and the retropatellar cartilage is seen in the upper part of the screen. The cartilage synovium junction is the landmark in this area of the joint **(Fig. 1)**.

Retropatellar Cartilage

The light cable is then rotated downward so that the scope then faces toward the retropatellar cartilage **(Fig. 2)**. The scope is swiped medially and laterally to inspect the medial and lateral patellar facets.

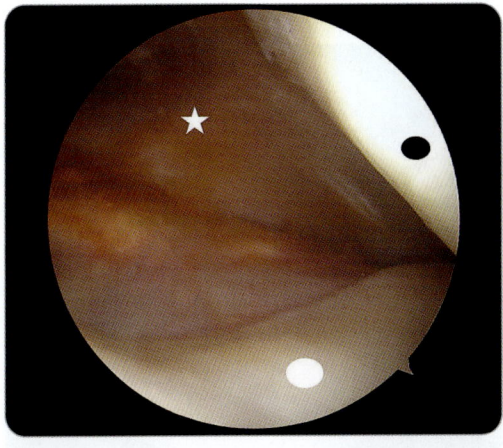

FIG. 1: Superior recess. Synovium (star), trochlea (white circle), and patellar cartilage (black circle).

Patellofemoral Joint

The patellofemoral articulation is then inspected **(Fig. 3)**. In cases with patellar dislocation, there may be a lateral patella tilt. Patellar tracking is then evaluated.

Lateral Recess and Capsule

With the knee in extension, the scope is then swiped along the lateral femoral condyle and the camera is then lifted up to enter the lateral recess. The medial and lateral recess is a common site for loose bodies in the joint and should always be evaluated **(Fig. 4)**. The popliteus tendon has an intra-articular insertion on the lateral femoral condyle just behind the lateral femoral cartilage and can be visualized. To visualize the popliteus tendon, the scope is advanced further into the lateral recess and the distal tendon can be seen inserted just behind the articular cartilage of the femur **(Fig. 5)**.

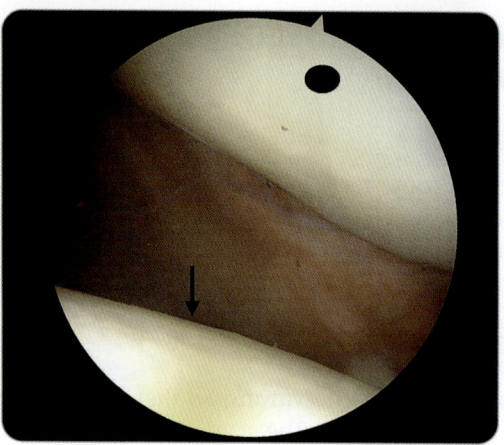

FIG. 2: Retropatellar cartilage (circle) and trochlea (arrow). Note the arrow is pointing up indicating the scope is facing upward.

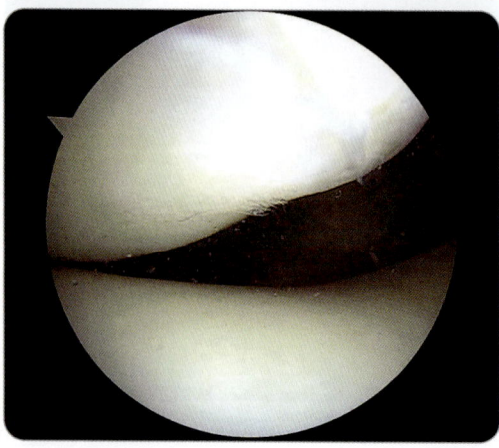

FIG. 3: Patellofemoral joint.

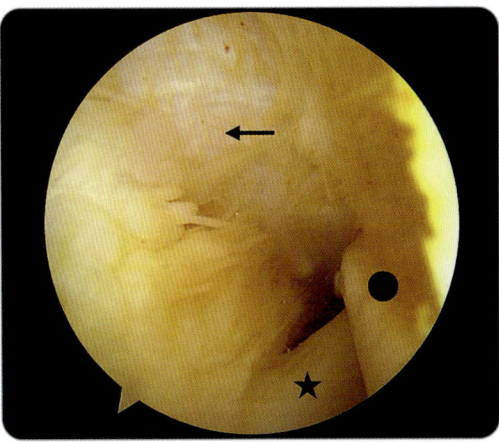

FIG. 4: Lateral recess. Lateral capsule (arrow), lateral femoral condyle (circle), and lateral tibial condyle (star).

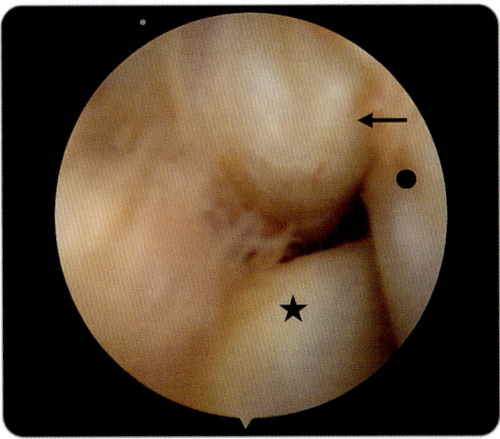

FIG. 5: Popliteus insertion (arrow), lateral femoral condyle (circle), and lateral tibial condyle (star).

Medial Recess and Capsule

After evaluating the lateral recess, the scope is then brought back into the superior recess. The same maneuver that was done to access the lateral recess is performed on the medial side to enter the medial recess **(Fig. 6)**.

Intercondylar Area

There are two ways to enter the joint from the superior recess.
1. The first is from the medial recess. With scope in the medial recess, the knee is flexed to 90°. The scope is then retracted and swiped in front of the medial femoral condyle to enter the notch.
2. The second way is from the superior recess. The scope is held in the center of the superior recess viewing the cartilage synovial junction of the superior

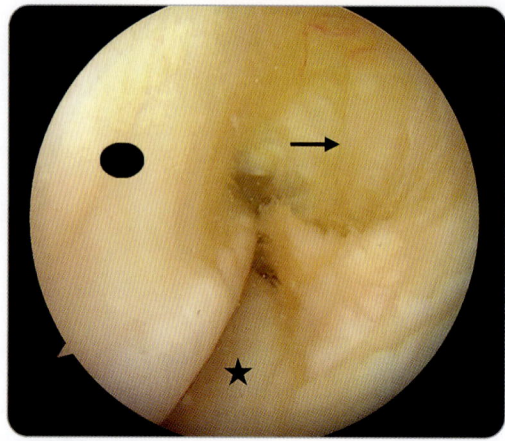

FIG. 6: Medial recess. Medial capsule (arrow), medial femoral condyle (circle), and medial tibial condyle (star).

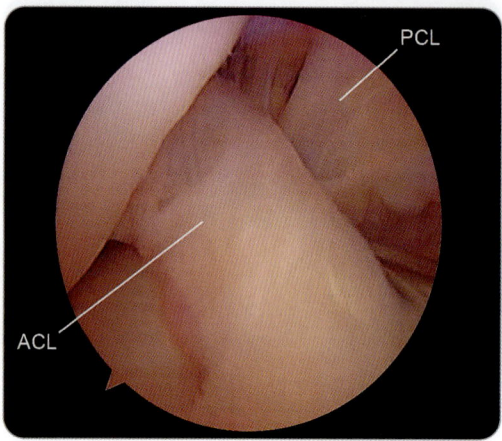

FIG. 7: Notch view showing anterior cruciate ligament (ACL) and posterior cruciate ligament (PCL).

recess. The knee is then gradually flexed and at the same time, the scope is slightly elevated to enter the notch.

The fat pad in the notch is cleared to visualize the anterior cruciate ligament (ACL) and posterior cruciate ligament (PCL) **(Fig. 7)**. There may be a band going from the roof of the notch to the front of the ACL called the ligamentum mucosum **(Fig. 8)**. This should not be mistaken for an ACL.

Lateral Compartment

The knee is placed in the figure-of-four position to enter the lateral compartment of the knee. Alternatively, the leg can be placed in varus to enter the knee cartilage. In cases where the surgeon is operating in the total knee replacement

CHAPTER 4: Diagnostic Round (Knee), Indications, and Contraindications

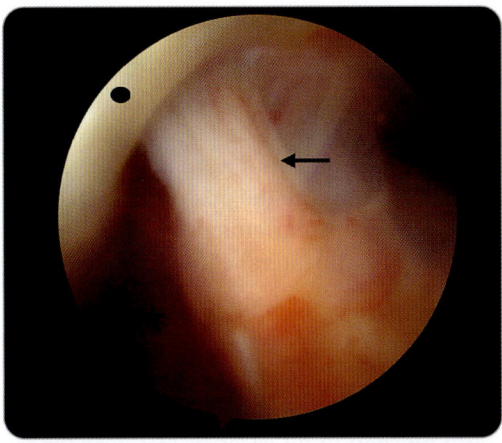

FIG. 8: Ligamentum mucosum (arrow), roof of the notch (circle), and lateral tibial condyle (star).

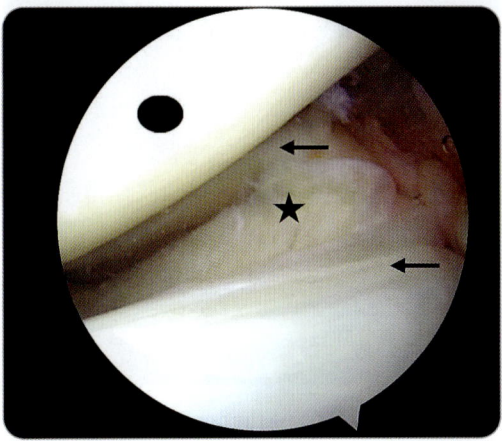

FIG. 9: Lateral compartment of knee. Anterior and posterior horn of lateral meniscus (arrows), lateral femoral condyle (circle), and lateral tibial condyle (star).

(TKR) position, just placing the leg flexed on the normal leg may open the lateral compartment allowing the surgeon to enter the lateral compartment. The lateral meniscus roots, body, and the attachment to the capsule is probed **(Fig. 9)**.

The lateral meniscus is not attached to the capsule in its entirety. There is a small opening in the capsular attachment to accommodate the popliteus tendon. This opening is called the popliteal hiatus. There is some mobility to the meniscus at the popliteal hiatus and this should not be diagnosed as a meniscus tear **(Fig. 10)**.

The cartilage of the lateral tibial and femoral condyle is inspected. The tibial cartilage can be seen by retracting the scope. Also, the cartilage underneath the body of the meniscus is inspected by lifting up the meniscus body. The femoral cartilage is then inspected. The entire femoral cartilage is inspected by flexing and extending the knee.

Medial Compartment

To visualize the medial compartment of the knee, the foot is placed in valgus and external rotation. The surgeon may place the leg on his own thigh to apply the valgus force or an assistant may be required to open the joint. The knee needs to be slightly flexed to visualize the posterior horn and body of the medial meniscus. Higher degrees of flexion will obscure the posterior meniscus. The body, anterior and posterior horn, and the capsular attachments of the medial meniscus are then probed **(Fig. 11)**. As with the lateral compartment, the medial femoral and tibial cartilage is inspected.

Posteromedial Compartment

The posteromedial compartment should always be inspected as it is a site for loose bodies. It should be seen in all cases of ACL tear for ramp tears. To enter

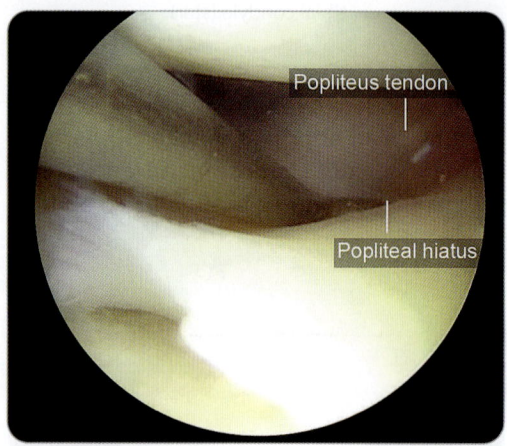

FIG. 10: Probing the popliteal hiatus.

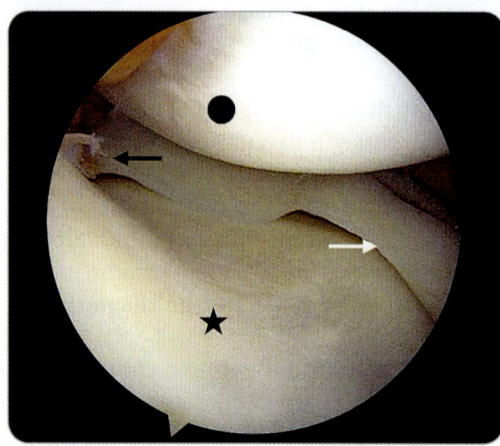

FIG. 11: Medial femoral condyle (circle), medial tibial condyle (star), posterior horn of medial meniscus (black arrow), and body of medial meniscus (white arrow).

the posteromedial compartment, the knee is in 90° flexion. The scope is taken in the space between the PCL and medial femoral condyle and external rotation force is applied **(Fig. 12)**. The scope is then gently pushed forward to enter the posteromedial compartment. In some cases, the fat pad in front of the PCL may be shaved to make space to enter the posteromedial compartment. Space can also be made between PCL and medial femoral condyle using a shaver keeping the mouth of the shaver facing the medial femoral condyle to avoid iatrogenic injury to PCL. The shaver creates a track after which it is easier to pass the scope in the tight space between PCL and medial femoral condyle. Once the scope enters the posteromedial compartment, an outside-in posteromedial portal can then be taken depending on the surgical procedure to be performed. One can visualize the posterior meniscus ramp and the posterior femoral condyle and posterior aspect of the medial meniscus from this vantage point **(Fig. 13)**.

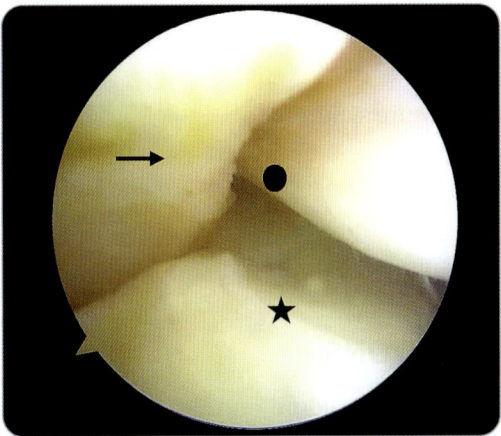

FIG. 12: Track to enter the posteromedial compartment is between the posterior cruciate ligament (PCL) (black arrow) and medial tibial condyle (black circle) with the knee in 90° flexion. Medial tibial condyle (star).

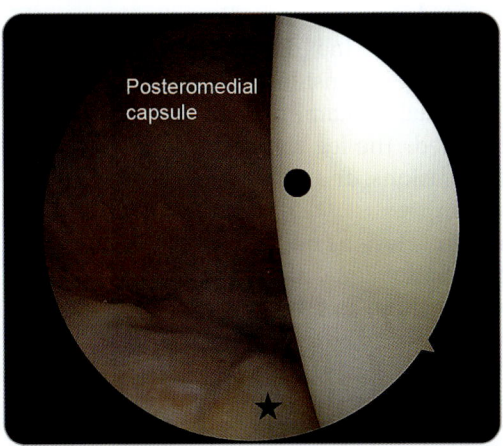

FIG. 13: Posteromedial compartment of knee. Medial femoral condyle (circle) and posterior horn of medial meniscus (star).

INDICATIONS

The indications for arthroscopy should be diagnosis oriented rather than symptom-oriented. Numerous clinical tests, radiographic studies, and if necessary, MRI can provide a definitive diagnosis, or at least narrow the differential diagnosis, in >95% of patients. There are a number of injuries and diseases that constitute an indication for arthroscopy:
- Meniscal lesions
- Cartilage lesions
- Recurrent joint effusions
- Limitation of motion
- Baker cysts
- Degenerative changes
- Loose bodies
- Osteochondral fractures
- Osteochondritis dissecans
- Patellar dislocation
- Excessive lateral pressure syndrome
- Plica syndrome
- ACL rupture
- PCL rupture
- Fractures
- Intra-articular infection

CONTRAINDICATIONS

Arthroscopy is an elective procedure and not a lifesaving operation, but still the patient should be in the best possible state of health condition. Coexisting systemic diseases (cardiac failure, hypertension, and diabetes mellitus) should be adequately controlled. If flulike symptoms are present, arthroscopy should be rescheduled. If the patient has a local infection with systemic manifestations [elevated WBC, elevated erythrocyte sedimentation rate (ESR), and malaise], the first priority is to eradicate the "distant" focus of infection. An intra-articular infection of the knee joint is considered an absolute and urgent indication for arthroscopy. The bacterial contamination of local skin areas on the operative limb should be excluded. The leg should be examined for pustules (pimples), folliculitis, old skin abrasions, and skin injuries caused by shaving of the leg (on the eve of the operation).

Any and all infectious lesions on the leg should contraindicate arthroscopy. An extensive capsuloligamentous injury with disruption of the posterior capsule is a relative contraindication, as it may cause substantial fluid leakage into the subcutaneous tissue during arthroscopy.

SUGGESTED READINGS

1. Strobel MJ (Ed). Manual of Arthroscopic Surgery. Berlin: Springer; 2002. p. 95.
2. Ward BD, Lubowitz JH. Basic knee arthroscopy part 3: diagnostic arthroscopy. Arthrosc Tech. 2013;2(4):e503-5.

Anterior Cruciate Ligament

*Aditya R Gunjotikar, Rohit Mahesh Sane,
Prasad Liladhar Chaudhari, Gaurav Kanade*

■ ANATOMY

The anterior cruciate ligament (ACL) arises from an elliptical area on the posteromedial aspect of the lateral femoral condyle. The ACL femoral attachment is behind the lateral intercondylar ridge (residents ridge) which runs on the medial aspect of lateral femoral condyle from proximal to distal till the articular cartilage. There is also the presence of a bifurcate ridge between the anteromedial and posterolateral bundle attachments **(Fig. 1)**. It passes forward, downward, and medially to the anterior intercondylar area of the tibia and inserts directly in front of the medial intercondylar tubercle. It is intimately attached to the anterior horn of the lateral meniscus. A study by Faretti and Fu showed the center of tibial ACL footprint to be 9 mm behind the intermeniscal ligament and 5 mm anterior to medial tibial spine **(Fig. 2)**.

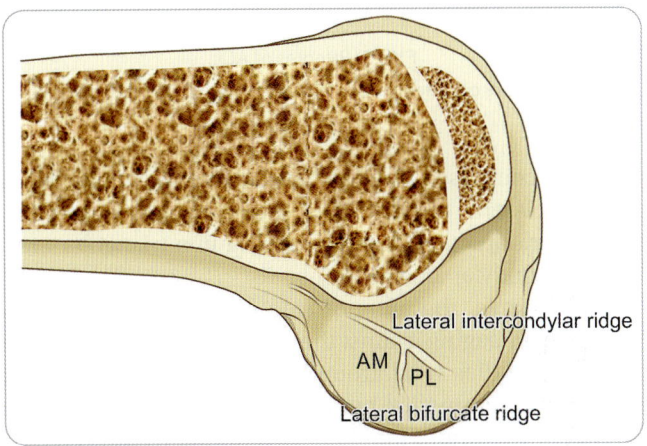

FIG. 1: Femoral attachment of ACL.
(ACL: anterior cruciate ligament)

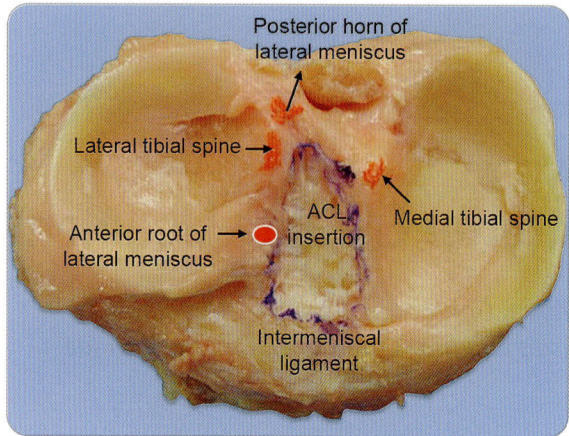

FIG. 2: Tibial ACL insertion site.
(ACL: anterior cruciate ligament)

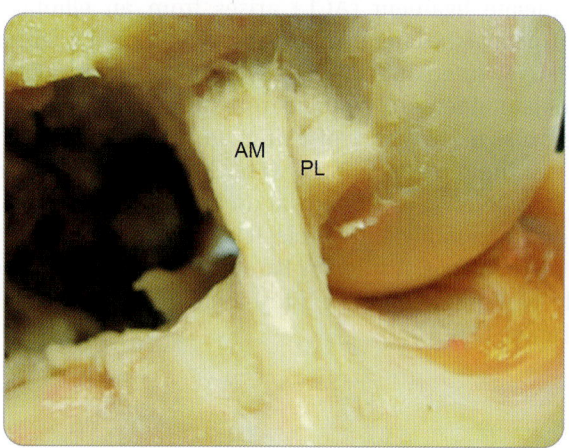

FIG. 3: Bundles of ACL.
(ACL: anterior cruciate ligament; AM: anteromedial; PL: posterolateral)

The ligament is composed of two fiber systems known as the anteromedial bundle and posterolateral bundle. These bundles intertwine in their approximately 2–2.5-cm intra-articular course, resulting in a triangular area of insertion in the anterior intercondylar area.

In the extended knee, the anterior side of the anteromedial bundle limits further extension by engaging against the roof of the intercondylar notch. As the knee is flexed, the bundles twist around each other, the posterolateral bundle rotates beneath the anteromedial bundle. The ligament loses its fan shape with increasing flexion and assumes the shape of a rounded cord **(Fig. 3)**.

Recognizing the anatomic course of the ACL bundles and their areas of attachment is of fundamental importance in ACL reconstructions.

CLINICAL DIAGNOSIS

The clinical diagnosis of an ACL rupture can be difficult but is simple if the examination is performed within a few hours of the injury. At this time, muscular guarding has not yet developed. An effusion (hemarthrosis) is often present. If a tense effusion is present, the joint cannot be examined.

The most sensitive clinical test for ACL injury is the Lachman test **(Fig. 4)**. A "stable" Lachman test is performed by placing the patient's thigh on the thigh of the examiner. While pressing the patient's thigh down against his own thigh, the examiner grasps the proximal lower leg and pulls it forward to test the amount of anterior tibial displacement and the quality of the endpoint.

The Lachman test has numerous advantages over the traditional anterior drawer test in 90° of flexion **(Fig. 5)**. Besides its high sensitivity for ACL rupture, it is only minimally affected by hemarthrosis. Even in acute injuries, it can be performed with relatively little pain, because the slightly flexed position relaxes the muscles about the knee. This position also permits greater anterior tibial translation in the presence of an isolated ACL rupture or a complex capsuloligamentous injury involving the ACL than when the knee is flexed 90°.

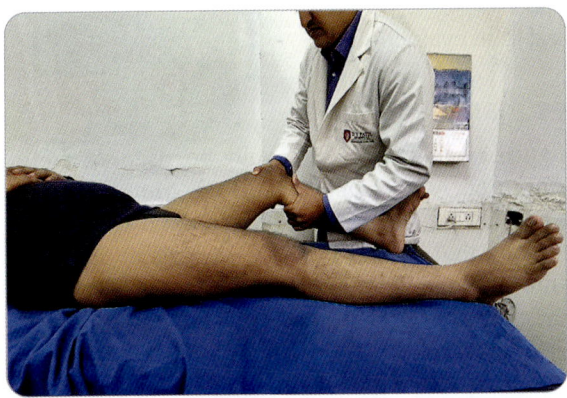

FIG. 4: Lachman test.

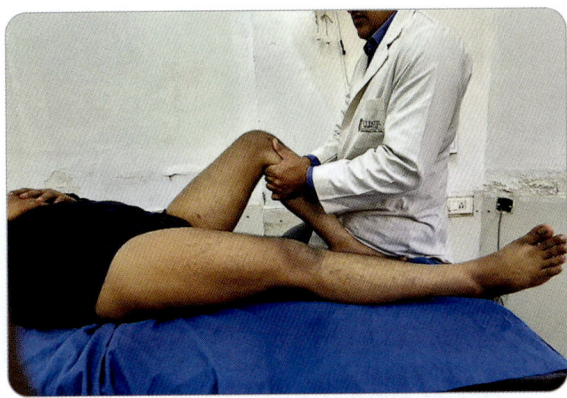

FIG. 5: Anterior drawer test.

The pivot shift test offers no advantages in acute injuries, and eliciting a dynamic anterior subluxation of the tibia frequently causes pain. Consequently, the various versions of the pivot shift test often yield a false-negative result in knees with an acute ACL injury.

In addition to the Lachman test, a dynamic anterior subluxation test, or pivot shift test, is also performed. Of the various pivot shift tests that are available, the "soft" pivot shift test has proven most satisfactory.

The clinical examination should also include tests for associated injuries (varus-valgus stress testing, point tenderness, and limits of motion).

The following tests are used in detecting associated injuries:
- Medial opening in extension and 30° of flexion (medial collateral ligament and posteromedial capsule)
- Lateral opening in extension and 30° of flexion (lateral collateral ligament and posterolateral capsule)
- *External rotation in 30° and 90° flexion*: The range of external rotation, combined with lateral opening in extension, gives information on the integrity of the posterolateral capsule. Whenever chronic instability is present, posterolateral components of the instability should be excluded.
- Meniscal tests
- Patellofemoral joint evaluation

Magnetic Resonance Imaging

Magnetic resonance imaging (MRI) should be used to confirm the clinical diagnosis of a ruptured ACL **(Figs. 6A and B)**. More than 90% of acute ACL ruptures can be reliably detected with the Lachman test.

It should be noted that MRI has few therapeutic implications, as it can only document the morphologic status of the joint; it is not useful for functional analysis. This is why, greater importance is placed on the clinical examination.

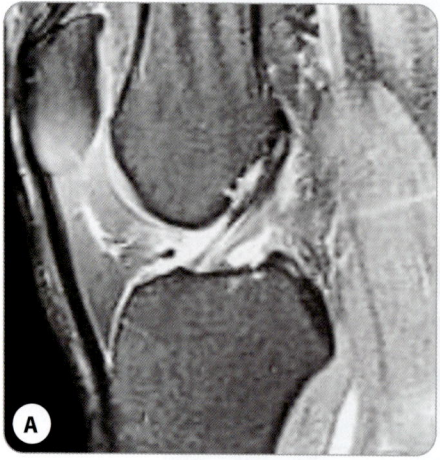 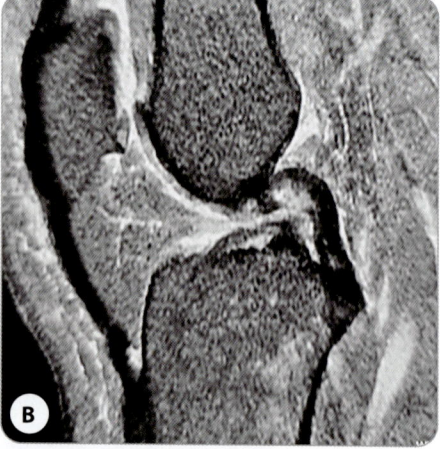

FIGS. 6A AND B: (A) Normal ACL; (B) Torn ACL.
(ACL: anterior cruciate ligament)

Magnetic resonance imaging can, however, detect associated injuries such as a lateral notch fracture and bone contusions or bruises, which most commonly involve the lateral limiting groove and the posterior third of the lateral tibial plateau in the ACL-injured knee.

■ TREATMENT

The following therapeutic approach is recommended for ACL ruptures: After the tear has been diagnosed, concomitant injuries that require immediate attention should be excluded. These injuries would include: rupture of the popliteus tendon, distal rupture of the medial collateral ligament, bucket-handle tear of the medial and/or lateral meniscus, and acute patellar dislocation.

These lesions can be detected or excluded by specific clinical tests, stress radiographs [posterior cruciate ligament (PCL) lesion], and MRI (PCL lesion and popliteus injury).

Nonoperative functional therapy is provided until the scheduled date of the ACL surgery. The nature of this therapy depends on the associated injuries. With a complete or partial tear of the medial collateral ligament, for example, the functional therapy is designed to promote healing of the ligament while avoiding immobilization-induced morbidity.

As a general rule, surgery is scheduled for 3–4 weeks after the knee injury. This allows sufficient time for healing of peripheral structures under a conservative treatment. It would be counterproductive to perform an ACL reconstruction 3 weeks after the injury if, for example, the medial collateral ligament is also torn. If the medial meniscus must be exposed during the surgery and a valgus stress must be applied to open up the medial joint space, this could seriously disrupt the healing of the medial collateral ligament.

As noted above, the joint should be free of irritation at the time of surgery. The treatment strategy depends on the patient's subjective complaints and the results of stability tests performed prior to surgery. Any of the three following situations may be found:

1. *Patient free of complaints*: Lachman test positive with a firm endpoint. Approximately, 10–15% of patients with an acutely torn ACL have a positive Lachman test with no endpoint immediately after the injury, but when examined "preoperatively" at 6–8 weeks, they show a positive Lachman test with a firm endpoint. This results from scar formation between the ruptured ACL and the lateral femoral condyle or PCL. While these scars do not have the same course as the ACL, they are often strong enough to stabilize the joint. If the patient is free of complaints, there is no need to proceed with arthroscopy. All the problems should be discussed with the patient in detail.
2. *Patient has pain and other complaints*: Lachman test positive with a firm endpoint. Arthroscopy is recommended to tailor further treatment to the intra-articular findings and the results of examination under anesthesia (pivot shift test?). If arthroscopy reveals intra-articular adhesions on the ACL and there is no sign of instability-related lesions, initial treatment may be limited to arthroscopic scar induction.
3. *Patient has pain and/or other complaints*: Lachman test positive with a soft endpoint. The patient is advised to have an ACL reconstruction.

Operative Technique

Routine steps in ACL reconstructions:
- Preparatory measure
- Diagnostic arthroscopy
- Graft harvesting
- Graft preparation
- Graft tensioning 80 N
- Femoral tunnel
- Tibial tunnel
- Femoral fixation (hybrid fixation)
- Impingement test
- Cycling of the graft
- Tibial fixation (hybrid fixation)
- Clearing the joint of debris
- Postoperative care

Preparatory Measure

Knee positioning, planning, and portals have to be spot on before intervening.

Diagnostic Arthroscopy

A diagnostic scopy is always initially done to confirm the diagnosis of ACL tear. The ACL may be torn in midsubstance, femoral or tibial insertion sites **(Fig. 7A)**. At times, the torn ACL stump may form a cyclops lesion **(Fig. 7B)** which may be painful and impinge in the notch. In chronic cases, there may be no ACL or a small portion of the ACL fibers remaining in the notch, the so-called empty notch sign **(Fig. 7C)**.

Sequence of arthroscopic examination during a diagnostic round has to be clear and in detail.
- Retropatellar cartilage
- Superior recess
- Femoropatellar joint
- Lateral recess and capsule
- Popliteal hiatus
- Medial recess and capsule
- Intercondylar area
- Lateral compartment
- Medial compartment
- Posteromedial compartment

Graft Harvesting

Depending on each case basis, and needs of the patient, an appropriate graft has to be harvested.

Graft Preparation

Regardless of whether the graft consists of the semitendinosus (ST) tendon, the ST and gracilis tendons, or a graft including a bone plug (central third of the

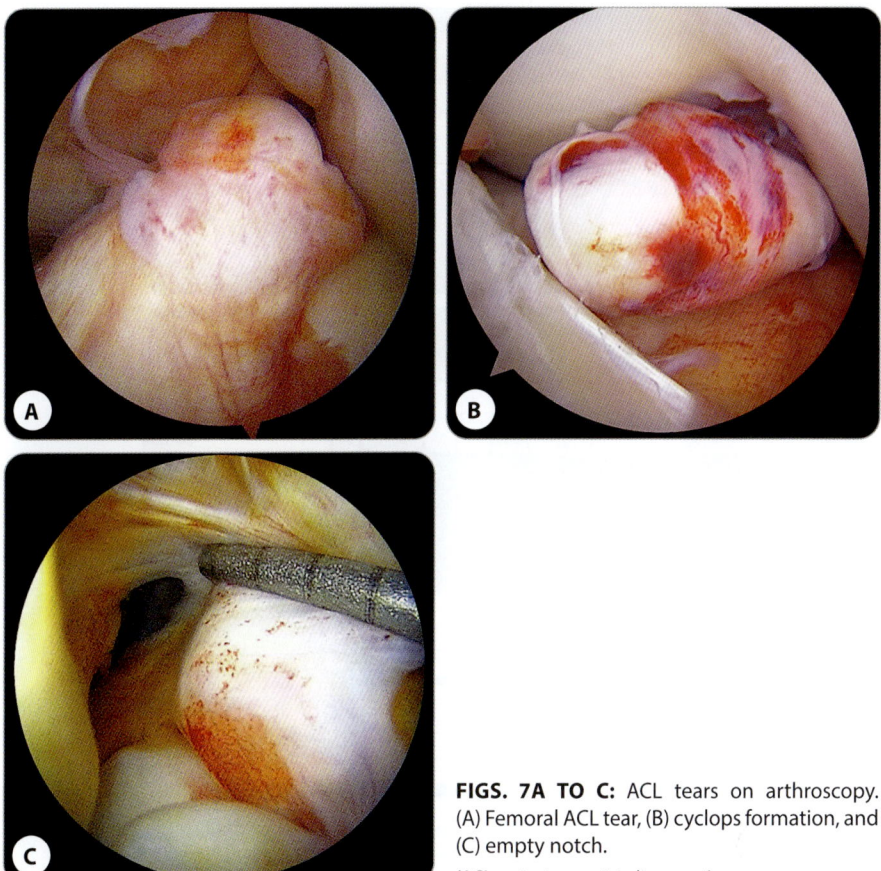

FIGS. 7A TO C: ACL tears on arthroscopy. (A) Femoral ACL tear, (B) cyclops formation, and (C) empty notch.

(ACL: anterior cruciate ligament)

patellar tendon and quadriceps tendon), it must first be cleaned of adherent fat and muscle fibers in preparation for use. The graft length and diameter should be determined with a sizer to determine the size of tunnels to be drilled **(Figs. 8A and B)**. The graft is then placed under tension on a graft board as the tunnels are drilled **(Fig. 8C)**.

Femoral Tunnel (Figs. 9A to F)

The femoral tunnel is carefully positioned to achieve isometric graft placement. Today, the concept of specific "isometric points" has been replaced by "isometric areas." This is a more accurate term when it is considered that the ACL is not a single cord or band but a complex ligamentous structure. Graft placement is assumed to be isometric when the distance between the tibial and femoral attachments changes by no more than 1.5–2 mm when the knee is moved from full extension to 90° of flexion. Experimental studies have shown that the isometric area is located approximately 5 mm posterosuperior to the center of the normal anatomic origin of the ACL. Thus, the standard over-the-top position provides a good reference point for isometric graft placement, and we use a femoral drill guide designed for use in the over-the-top position.

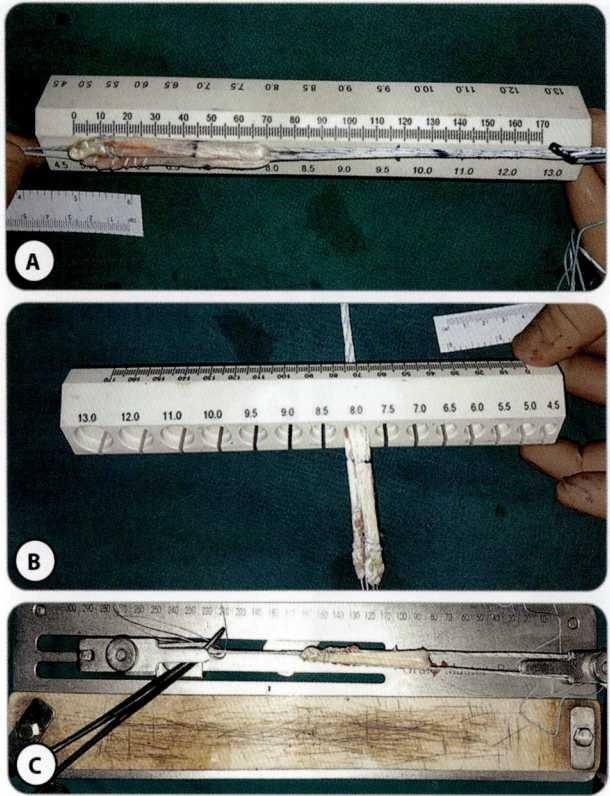

FIGS. 8A TO C: Prepared graft. (A) Measuring graft length, (B) Measuring graft diameter, and (C) Graft under tension on graft board.

Tunnel placement through medial instrument portal: The tunnel is placed through the medial instrument portal, which must be positioned accordingly. It can be difficult to reach the over-the-top position through a very high medial portal, even with maximum knee flexion. Thus, the medial instrument portal should be placed at a lower (suprameniscal) level. This may involve some damage to the infrapatellar fat pad. This placement technique results in a more laterally directed femoral tunnel. Maximum knee flexion (>120°) is necessary to reach the over-the-top position at the back of the lateral femoral condyle. A desired tunnel length and diameter is then sequentially drilled **(Fig. 2)**.

Tibial Tunnel (Figs. 10A to D)

A constant and reliable reference point for positioning the tibial tunnel is the anterior circumference of the PCL, and just posterior to the anterior horn of the lateral meniscus. With the knee in 90° of flexion, the center of the tibial footprint of the ACL is consistently located 7 mm anterior to the anterior circumference of the PCL. This distance does not vary with the size of the knee joint.

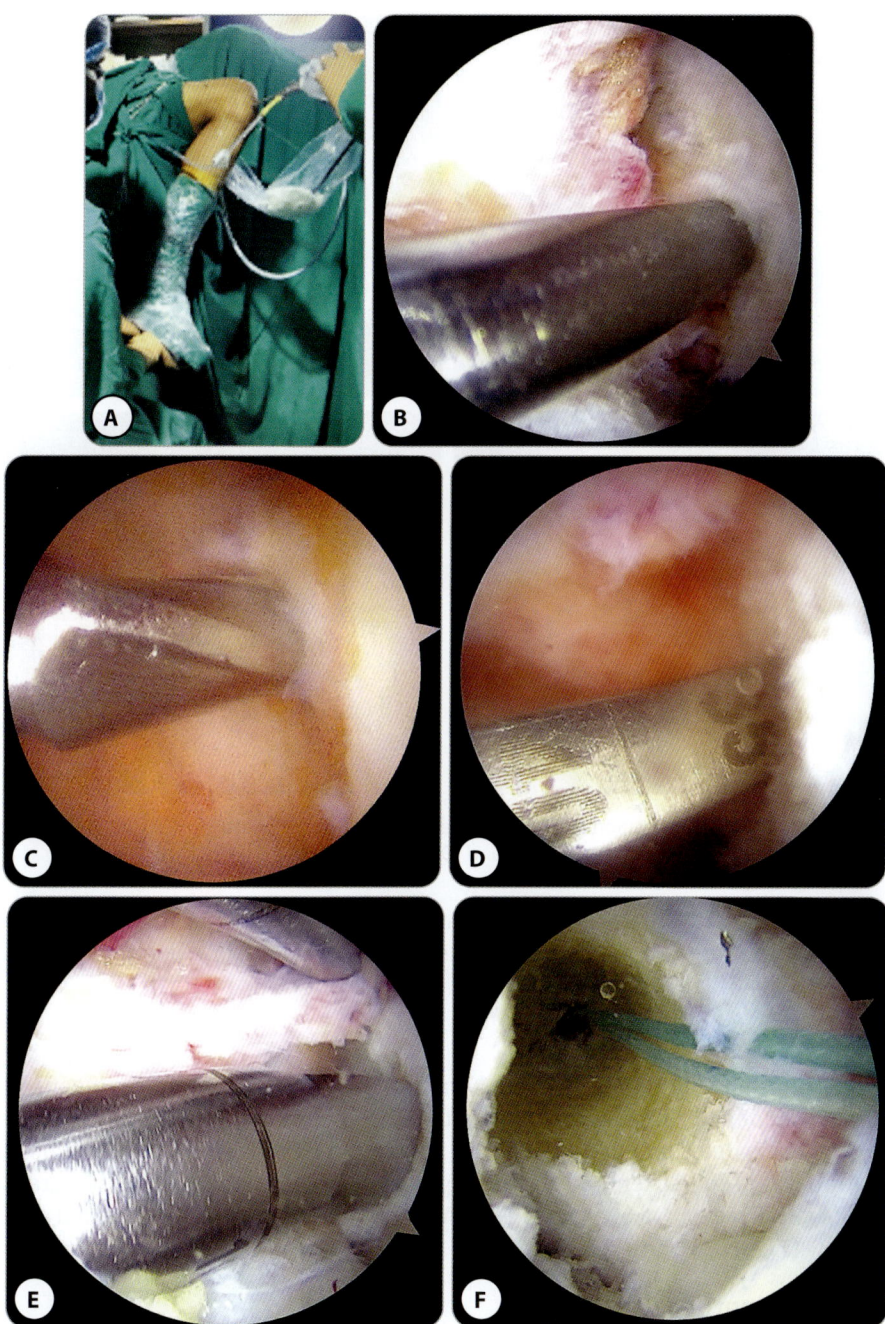

FIGS. 9A TO F: (A) Hyperflexion of knee to drill femoral tunnel, (B) Drilling with a beath pin, (C) Drilling 4.5-mm tunnel, (D) Measuring the 4.5 femoral tunnel, (E) Drilling the final tunnel, and (F) Final funnel position.

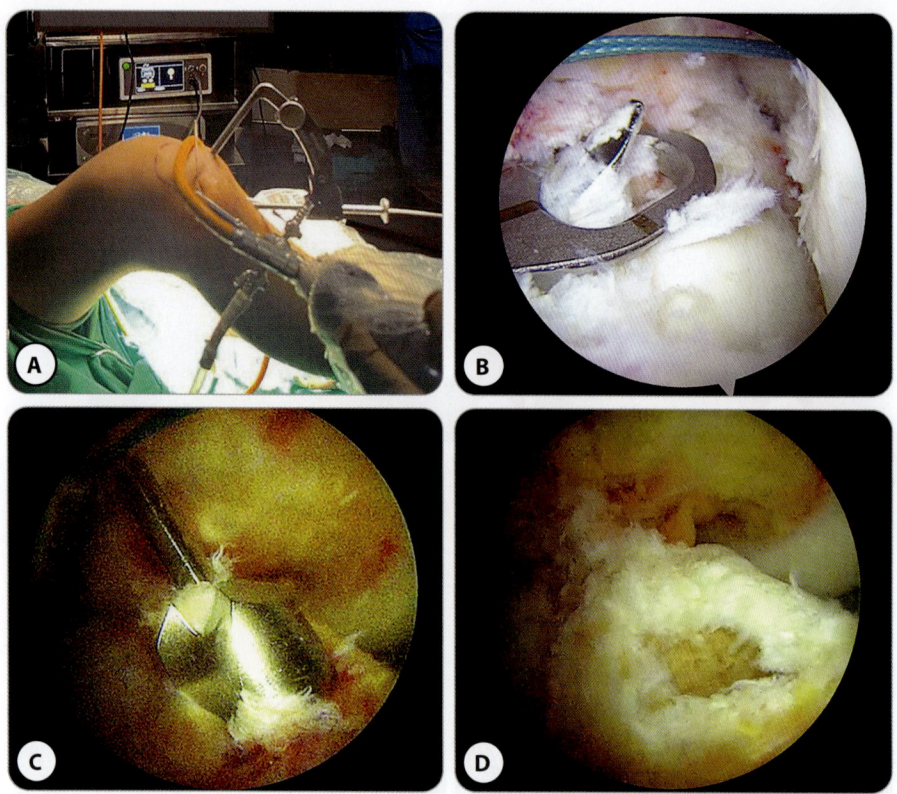

FIGS. 10A TO D: (A) Position and jig placement, (B) Drilling the beath pin, (C) Final tunnel drilling, and (D) Final tunnel.

The tibial drill guide is inserted and positioned directly in front of the anterior circumference of the PCL. A desired tunnel length and diameter is then sequentially drilled **(Fig. 2)**.

Femoral Fixation

When a fixation button is used, the graft is linked to the button by means of threads, a looped thread, etc. The length of the construct that links the button to the graft is determined mainly by the length of the femoral tunnel. The type of graft that is used (ST tendon, BTB) is significant in this regard. Soft tissue grafts are usually fixed with a button **(Figs. 11A to C)** whereas bony grafts are fixed with a screw **(Fig. 12)**.

Impingement Test

While tension is placed on the grafts, the knee is taken through approximately 30 cycles of complete flexion and extension **(Fig. 6)**. This not only helps to align the grafts but also tests for impingement between the grafts and bony structures (intercondylar roof, lateral femoral condyle). If necessary, the notchplasty is extended. This must be done very carefully after graft passage, preferably using a small chisel. The area is then smoothed with a fine rasp.

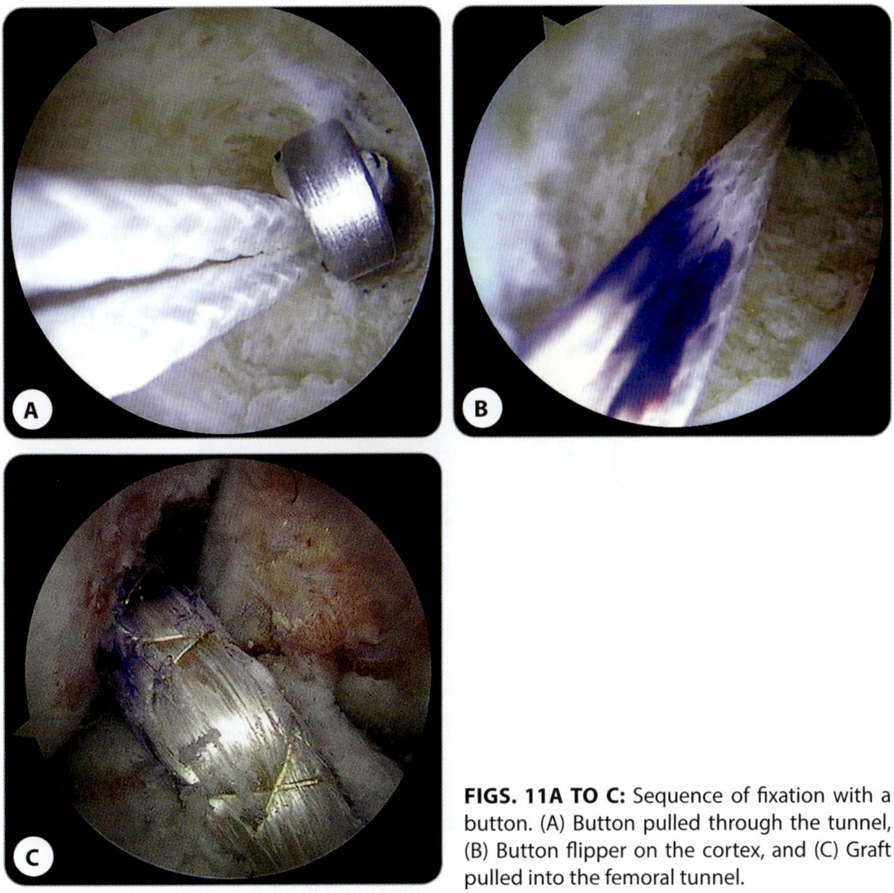

CHAPTER 5: Anterior Cruciate Ligament

FIGS. 11A TO C: Sequence of fixation with a button. (A) Button pulled through the tunnel, (B) Button flipper on the cortex, and (C) Graft pulled into the femoral tunnel.

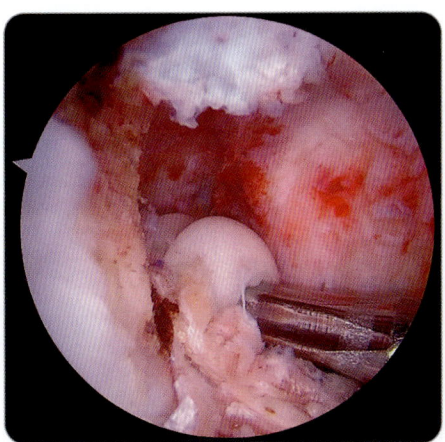

FIG. 12: Femoral fixation of ACL graft with a Bioscrew.
(ACL: anterior cruciate ligament)

The impingement test is difficult to interpret if a large ACL stump has been left in place or if the ACL remnant has been hollowed out and retained as a synovial stump **(Fig. 13)**.

Tibial Fixation

The type of tibial fixation depends on the length of the graft. An interference screw is used in cases where the graft is at the mouth of the tunnel whereas a suture disk is used in cases where the graft is not present at the mouth of the tunnel.

Keeping the graft under tension, knee in 30° of flexion, and a posterior drawer force application, is the right way to have a tibial fixation **(Figs. 14A and B)**.

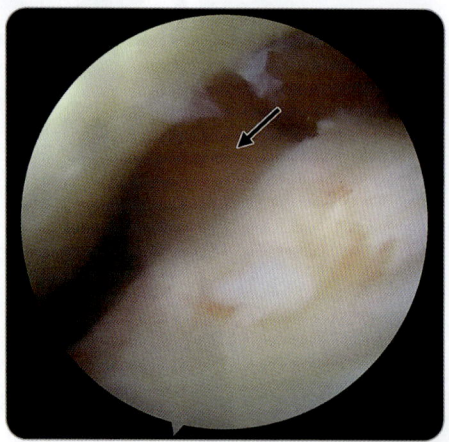

FIG. 13: No impingement of the graft on full extension. Arrow: ACL graft between femoral and tibial condyles while the knee is in full extension.
(ACL: anterior cruciate ligament)

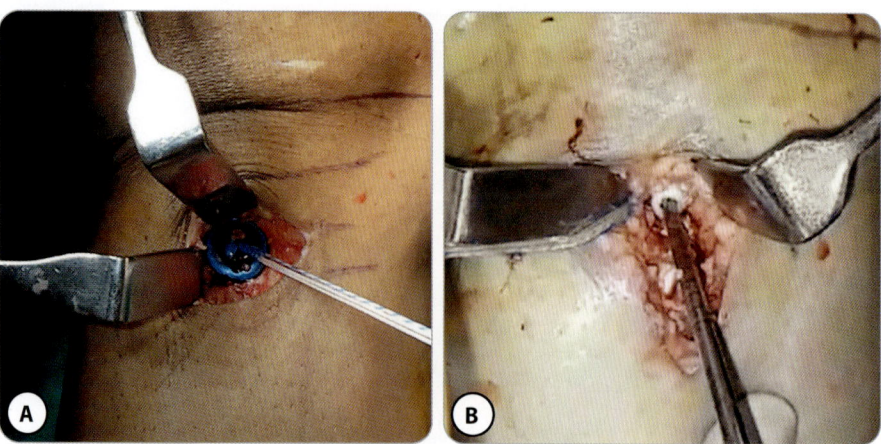

FIGS. 14A AND B: Tibial fixation of ACL graft. (A) Endobutton fixation, and (B) Bioscrew fixation.
(ACL: anterior cruciate ligament)

Clearing the Joint of Debris

Before the operation is concluded, the entire joint cavity is cleaned of debris. The drilling and smoothing can generate cancellous bone fragments of varying size, which are often scattered throughout the joint. They can be removed with an irrigation cannula or motorized instrument (shaver), but the latter should be used carefully to avoid sucking portions of the graft and synovium into the cutting port. The irrigation cannula should also be passed into the posterolateral and posteromedial recesses of the joint. The medial and lateral compartments are also cleaned. The suprapatellar pouch should also be inspected and cleared of any cancellous bone debris.

Postoperative Care

Postoperative care is dependent on the type of surgery done, the associated lesions, and demographics of the patient. A general care of the wound and leg should be done. The knee should be placed in a long knee brace with protected weight bearing.

SUGGESTED READINGS

1. Strobel MJ. Manual of arthroscopic surgery. Berlin: Springer; 2002. pp. 367-75.
2. Ferretti M, Doca D, Ingham SM, Cohen M, Fu FH. Bony and soft tissue landmarks of the ACL tibial insertion site: an anatomical study. Knee Surg Sports Traumatol Arthrosc. 2011;20(1): 62-8.
3. Ferretti M, Ekdahl M, Shen W, Fu FH. Osseous Landmarks of the Femoral Attachment of the Anterior Cruciate Ligament: An Anatomic Study. Arthroscopy. 2007;23(11):1218-25.

Meniscus

Bhushan Jaywantrao Patil, Sandeep Narayan Deore,
Prasad Liladhar Chaudhari, Sushmit Singh

■ INTRODUCTION

Meniscus is a crescent-shaped wedge of fibrocartilage located in the medial and lateral compartment of the knee joint. Lateral compartment is smaller than the medial but the lateral meniscus covers almost 80% articular surface and medial meniscus covers 60% of the articular surface. Peripheral circumferential fibers of the meniscus contain type I collagen and have high tensile strength which helps in distributing the hoop stresses. Shock absorption and load distribution are the important function of the menisci. Forces sustained by menisci in different knee angles differ being maximum forces at the maximum knee flexion. Posterior horn of the medial meniscus also resists anterior translation of tibia providing stability. Radial tear in any of the meniscus especially in the posterior horn medial meniscus (root tear) is devastating injury which causes 200–300% increase in load of the joint and may lead to rapid progression of arthritis.

■ BLOOD SUPPLY

A perimeniscal capillary plexus is formed by the blood vessels that arise from the lateral, middle, and medial geniculate arteries and penetrate through the joint capsule. Here, the radial branches enter the menisci and supply the peripheral quarter of the menisci (red zone). It is noted in cadaveric studies that the radial branches penetrate the menisci to a depth of 2–3 mm, with the most consistent blood supply occurring at the posterior and anterior horns. The posterolateral aspect of the lateral meniscus, adjacent to the popliteus tendon, is avascular, as is the white zone of the meniscus. Cooper described these zones by dividing the meniscus into three radial sections (zone A, B, and C) from posterior to anterior and the width into three from peripheral to central.

In addition, the blood supply to the menisci varies with age. By the age of 20, blood vessels are only present in the peripheral third, which further regresses to a quarter at the age of 50.

SYMPTOMS

Acute traumatic meniscal injury is seen in a younger individual and degenerative meniscus injury in middle-aged patients. Many patients give a history of a rotational knee injury. Others describe a sudden tearing sensation and sharp pain after squatting. Meniscal tears may also cause intermittent locking, snapping, or limitation of extension. Older meniscal lesions are frequently associated with a serous effusion and quadriceps atrophy. There may also be a constant or intermittent block to knee extension. Acute meniscal tears are predominantly associated with acute trauma symptoms, hemarthrosis, and possible accompanying capsuloligamentous injuries [torn collateral ligament and ruptured anterior cruciate ligament (ACL)]. Many patients present with a locked knee (bucket handle tear) with previous knee injury suggestive of old ACL tear.

CLINICAL EVALUATION

Clinically, the most relevant sign is jointline tenderness. Range of movement may be restricted in acute tears due to locked meniscus fragment hemarthrosis. Commonly done test is McMurray's Test with different rotations for medial and lateral meniscus. Apley's grinding test done in a prone position is more painful in acute injuries. Chronic tears may present with joint line tenderness and near normal knee movement. Meniscus posterior root tears usually present with posterior knee pain which increases on hyperextension. Lateral meniscus discoid pattern present at younger age with snapping or clicking during mid flexion to extension (**Figs. 1 and 2**).

MENISCAL TEAR PATTERNS

Meniscus tears are classified according to anatomic location and therefore proximity to blood supply and also tear morphology. Depending upon vascularity, meniscus tears are classified into peripheral red–red zone, middle red–white zone and central white–white zone with decreasing vascularity from periphery toward center. Depending upon tear geometry, they are classified into longitudinal, bucket handle tears, radial tears, horizontal, and combination

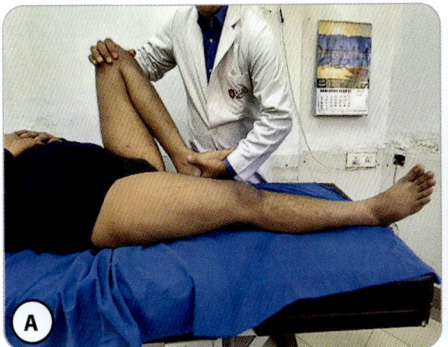 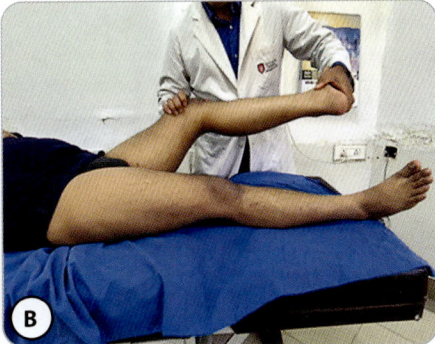

FIGS. 1A AND B: McMurray's test for medial meniscus.

of these **(Figs. 3 and 4A to C)**. Other patterns are Posterior horn root tears and RAMP tears (meniscocapsular junction tears) **(Fig. 5)**.

Stability and sporting activity are one of the few factors that characterize the tears. The pattern of meniscal injuries in the ACL-deficient knee is similar in both children and adults. A higher non-progressive incidence of lateral meniscal tears occurs acutely, and a lower increasing rate of medial tears occurs chronically.

Vertical type of tear is the most common to be repaired. They are mostly full thickness and may be unstable (bucket handle). They usually occur in trauma and are associated with ACL injuries. They are often extensive.

The effects of radial tears depend on whether they are incomplete or complete. Incomplete tears start centrally and do not reach the intact peripheral rim; the circumferential collagen fibers of the meniscus remain intact thus stability remains. Small incomplete radial tears, which are in the white–white zone, are often treated with partial meniscectomy. This contrasts with complete radial tears which traverse the circumferential collagen fibers resulting in extrusion of the meniscus and abnormal load transmission which is equivalent to total meniscectomy.

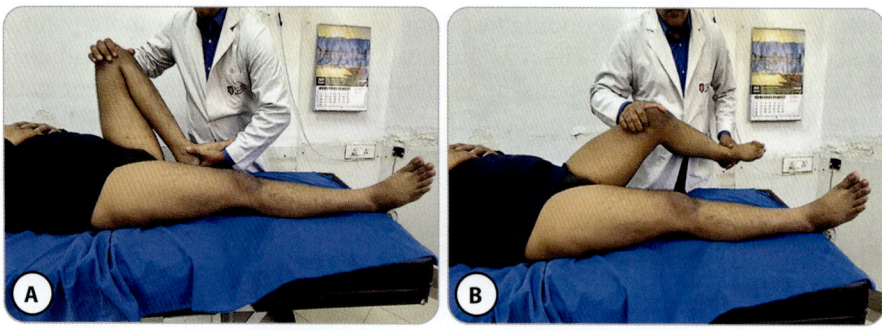

FIGS. 2A AND B: McMurray's test for lateral meniscus.

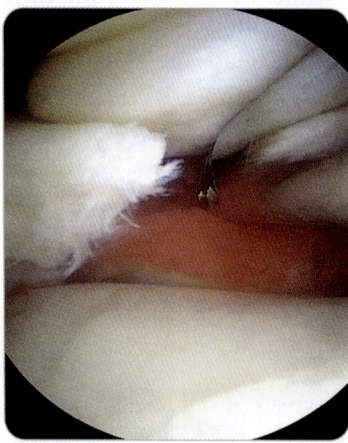

FIG. 3: Radial tear of lateral meniscus.

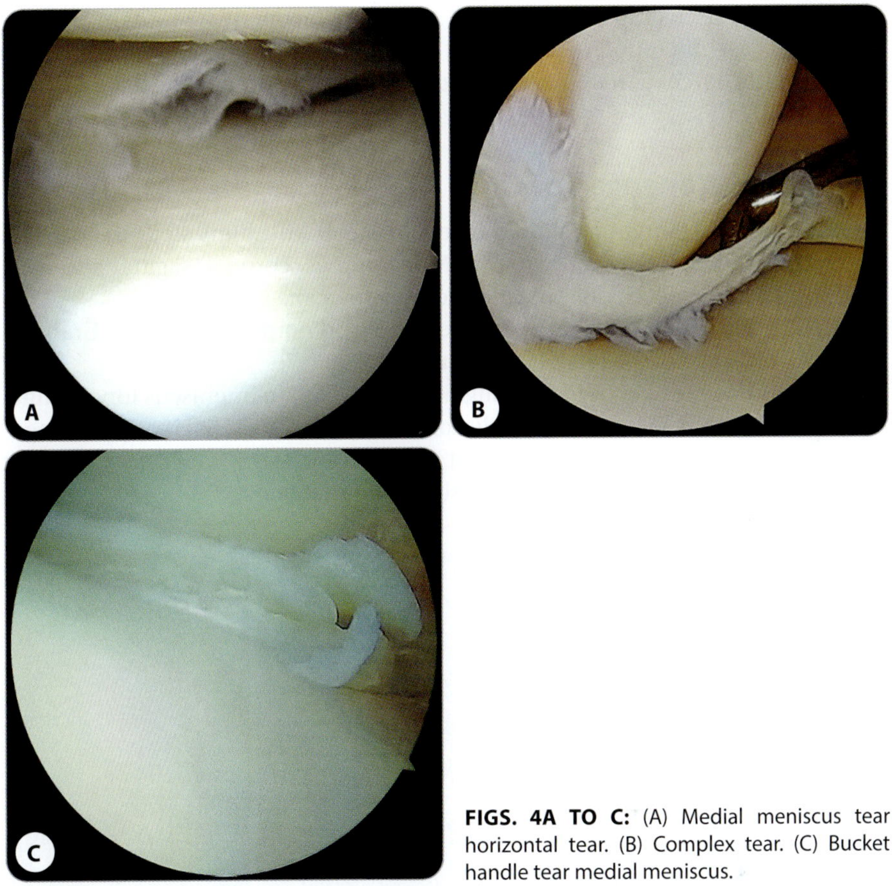

FIGS. 4A TO C: (A) Medial meniscus tear horizontal tear. (B) Complex tear. (C) Bucket handle tear medial meniscus.

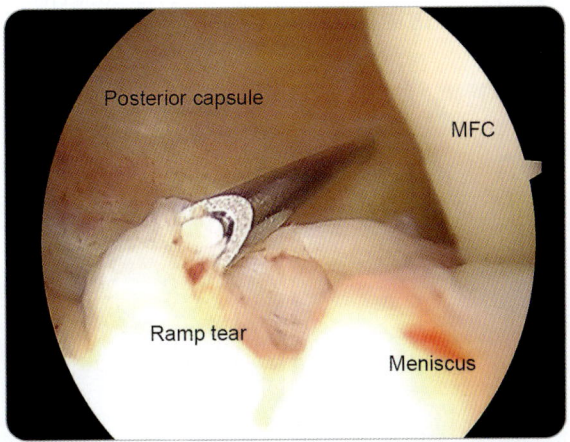

FIG. 5: Ramp tear at meniscocapsular junction.

Lateral meniscus radial tear is seen along with acute ACL injury in a young patient. In case of complete radial tear grade III and IV, there are tremendous increase in the forces across the lateral compartment leading to cartilage changes and early arthritis.

Magnetic Resonance Imaging

We as Orthopedic Surgeons should be able to read MRI films so as to correlate patients clinical presentation with the MRI findings, coronal, sagittal and axial T2 images help in identifying specific geometry of tear.

Grade I and Grade II signal in the meniscus and normal signal, and Grade III signal is suggestive of the tear **(Figs. 6 and 7)**.

Coronal images help in identifying medial and lateral meniscus longitudinal tears, horizontal cleavage tears and discoid lateral meniscus. Sagittal MRI images help in diagnosing posterior horn root tears (Ghost sign), radial tears, bucket handle longitudinal tears (double PCL sign) and root tears.

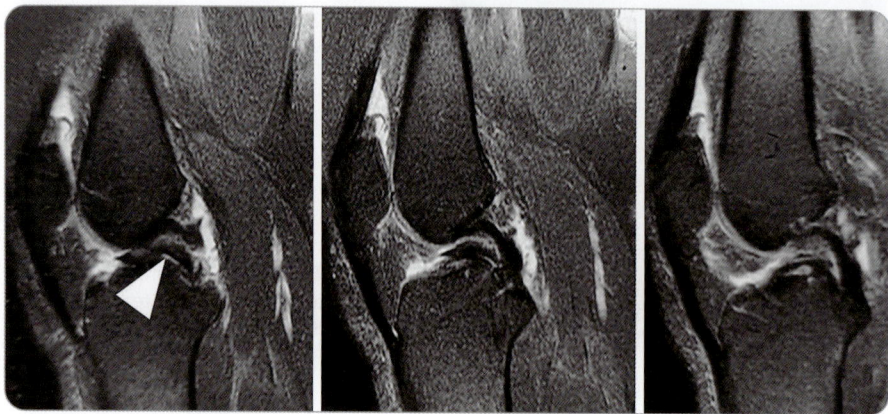

FIG. 6: Double posterior cruciate ligament (PCL) sign for bucket handle medial meniscus tear in sagittal MRI cuts (arrowhead).

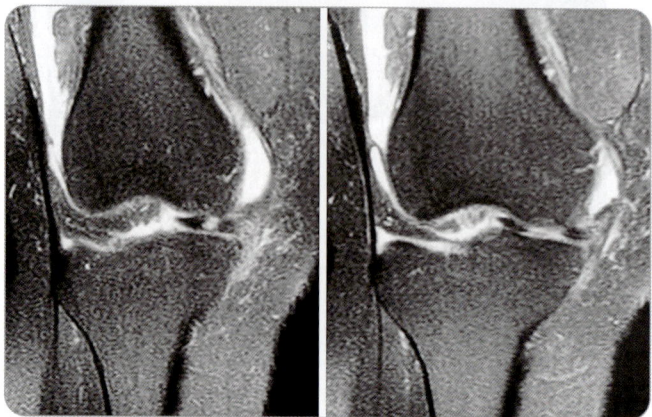

FIG. 7: Longitudinal tear medial meniscus in coronal MRI cuts.

TREATMENT

Treatment depends on the morphologic status of the meniscus as determined by arthroscopy, the correlation of clinical and arthroscopic findings. Various treatment options are available: resection, repair, combination of resection and repair, freshening the lesion, and nontreatment.

Resection

Meniscal resection is most commonly performed. It involves the removal of unstable, torn, degenerative, or heavily scarred areas of meniscal tissue. Various techniques are available for meniscal resection: piecemeal removal, en-bloc resection, combined piecemeal, and en-bloc resection. Visualization of the meniscus is the key during knee arthroscopic procedure. Adequate opening of medial and lateral compartments is necessary to pass the cutting instruments without damaging the cartilage. For medial compartment visualization knee is held in extension, external rotation and valgus force is given by the surgeon's waist or the assistant. Still more opening can be done by pie-crusting of the MCL at femoral or tibial attachment with no. 18 needle (**Figs. 8A and B**).

For lateral compartment visualization, knee is held in figure-of-4 position (**Fig. 9**).

Repair

Given the essential function of the menisci in protecting the articular cartilage, it is best to try and repair a torn meniscus whenever possible. Regardless of the fixation technique that is used, the repair includes two basic steps: (1) freshening the tear and (2) repairing the tear.

Techniques of Freshening the Meniscus to Stimulate Biology

Because meniscal fibrocartilage is a bradytrophic tissue, the tear site should be freshened to promote healing. Several techniques are available: debridement, needling, trephination, perimeniscal synovectomy, microfracture in the femoral notch and fibrin clot or platelet rich plasma (PRP).

Repair Techniques

Various repair techniques have been described in recent years. The technique of choice in a given case depends on various factors: location of the lesion, type of lesion (longitudinal tear, bucket-handle tear, ramp lesion, or horizontal tear), stability that the repair can achieve, time needed for the repair, available instrumentation, cost of the repair instruments and implants, and individual operator preference.

The three basic techniques for arthroscopic meniscal repairs are: (1) all-inside technique, (2) inside-out technique, and (3) outside-in technique.

All-inside Technique

In this technique, the needle is inserted into the meniscus from within the joint and also exits the meniscal tissue inside the joint. The all-inside technique is

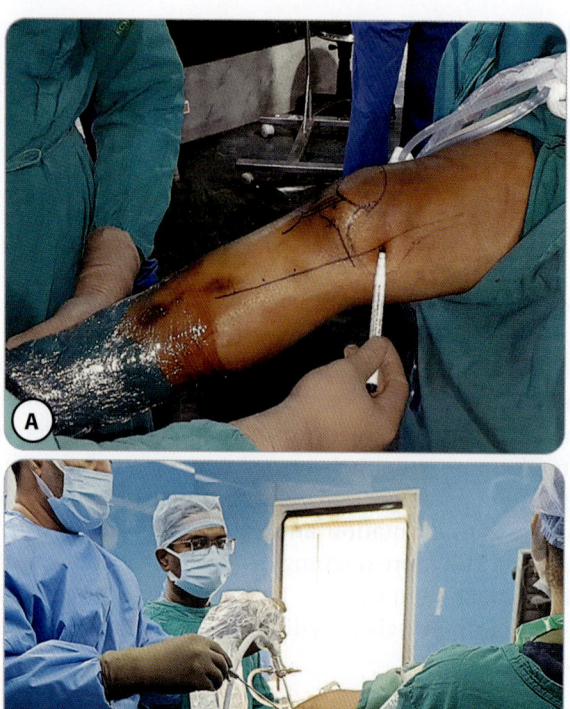

FIGS. 8A AND B: (A) Clinical landmark for medial collateral ligament (MCL) pie-crusting. (B) Valgus stress in extension by surgeon's waist.

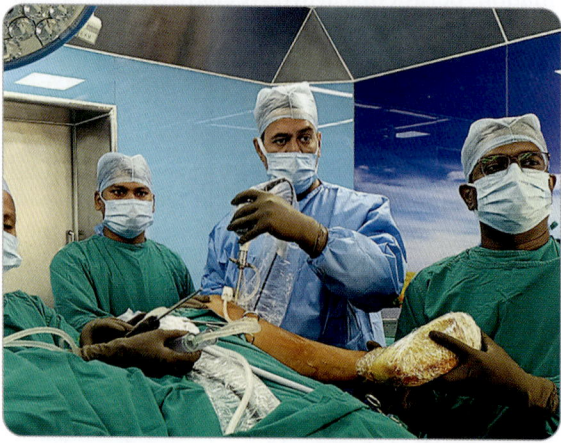

FIG. 9: Figure-of-4 position for lateral meniscus.

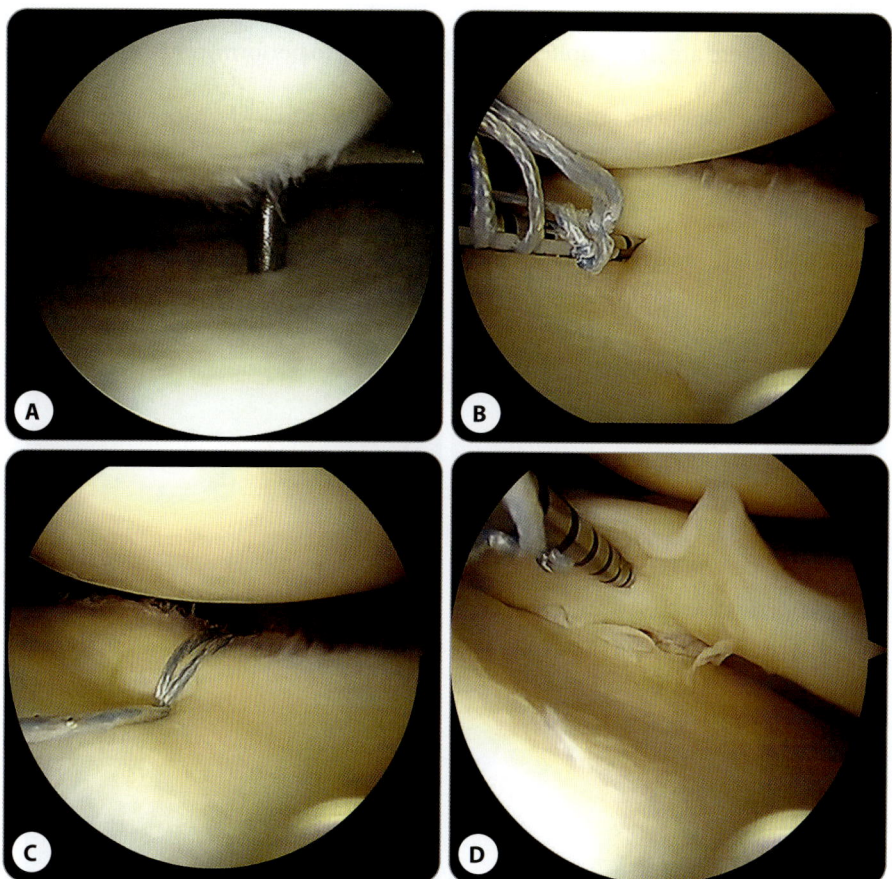

FIGS. 10A TO D: (A) After MCL pie crusting. (B) All-inside meniscus implant on needle being passed, (C) tightening of the knot. (D) Undersurface of meniscus being repaired.

useful for repairing posterior third meniscal tears that are difficult to access with other techniques **(Figs. 10A to D)**.

Inside-out Technique (Fig. 11)

In this technique, a needle is introduced through the instrument portal and is passed through the displaced meniscal fragment from inside the joint and through the intact meniscal rim. It is then brought out through the capsule and subcutaneous tissue. Because the needle may be difficult to direct, guide cannulas have been developed. Since this technique can be used for posterior meniscal repairs, one guide cannula is not sufficient, and assorted curved cannulas must be used.

Outside-in Technique

In an outside-in repair, sutures are passed from outside to inside the joint. This technique is the most widely utilized because of its many advantages, and it can be used in various meniscal segments **(Fig. 12)**.

Advantages:
- *Simple*: There are no complicated surgical steps to perform, and the technique is easy to learn.
- *Fast*: An experienced surgeon performs the repair quickly. More time may be required in anatomically complex situation.

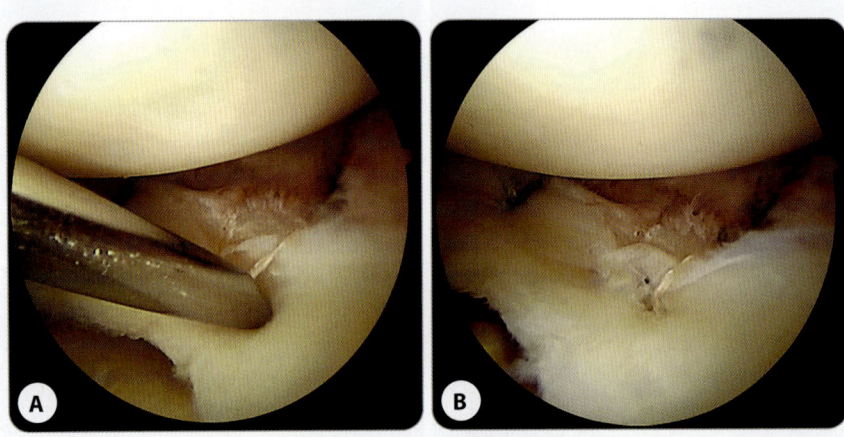

FIGS. 11A AND B: Inside-out repair of medial meniscus.

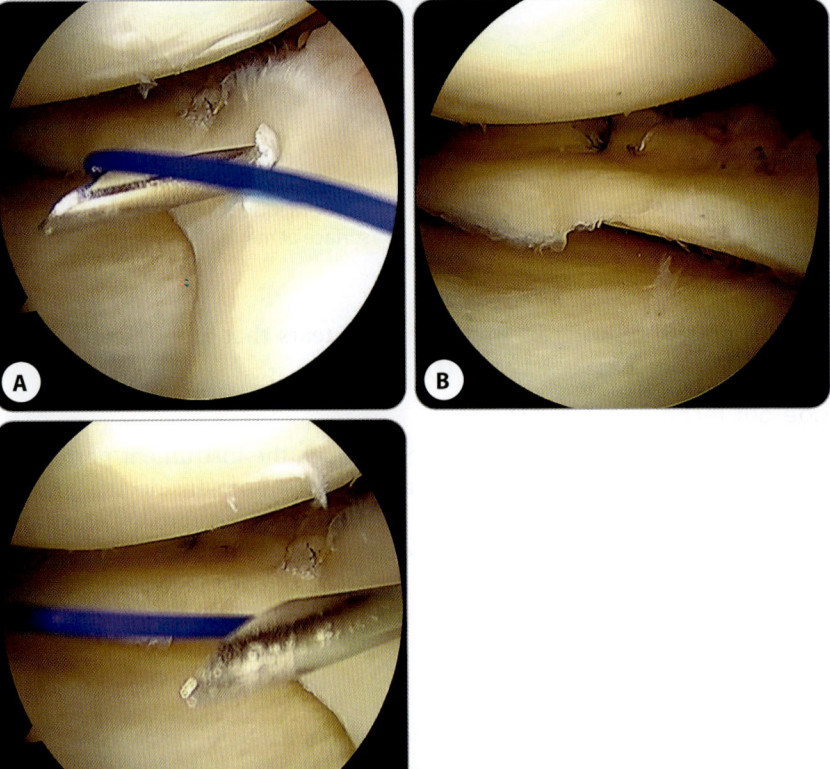

FIGS. 12A TO C: Outside-in repair of anterior third of medial meniscus.

- *Safe*: Because the technique is simple, complications and problems rarely arise.
- *Low cost*: A number of companies offer meniscal repair sets, but the technique can be performed with "ordinary" hypodermic needles or spinal needles.

Disadvantage:
Limited applications: It cannot be used to repair tears located in the posterior third of the medial or lateral meniscus.

Indications:
The outside-in technique is best for repairing tears within the anterior horn (anterior third) or middle third of the medial or lateral meniscus. The popliteus tendon forms the lateral boundary. Lesions anterior to the tendon are amenable to an outside-in repair. Lesions posterior to the tendon should be repaired using the all-inside technique.

Repair of Horizontal Meniscus Tear

Horizontal cleavage (intrasubstance) tears extend parallel to the tibial plateau, dividing the meniscus longitudinally. They tend to occur as part of a degenerative process and may be accompanied by a meniscal cyst and may exist without clinical symptoms. Symptomatic tears need surgical management in the form of partial meniscectomy and sometimes stabilizing vertical sutures to the periphery **(Figs. 13A and B)**.

Combined Resection and Repair

In young patients or patients with a large tear fragment in the lateral meniscus, one option is to combine a partial meniscectomy with meniscal repair. With a large, peripheral bucket handle tear of the lateral meniscus in which the fragment is very difficult or impossible to reduce, one should consider the option of combining resection and repair. For example, the lateral meniscus may be detached at the anterior horn so that the tear can be reduced, and then the posterior two-thirds of the meniscus is repaired.

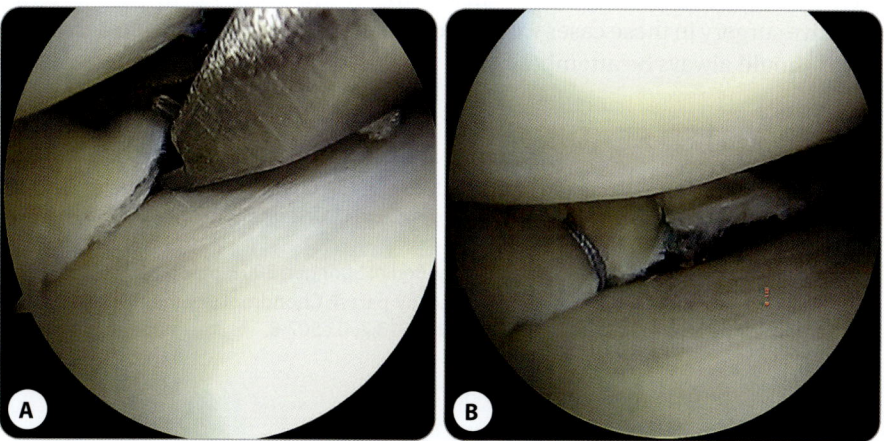

FIGS. 13A AND B: All-inside repair of horizontal cleavage tear with knee scorpion device.

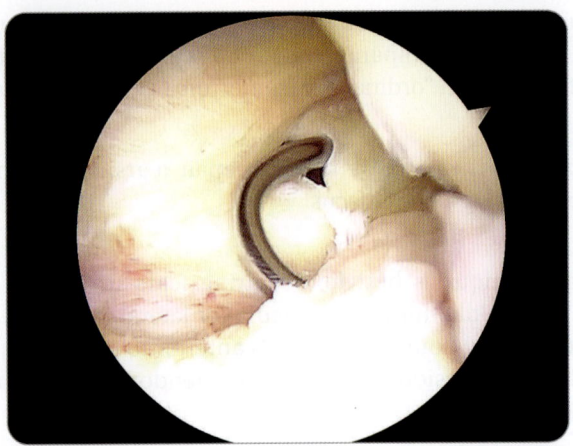

FIG. 14: Ramp repair with retrograde suture passing device ACCU-PASS.

Freshening the Tear

Incomplete tears (<1.5 cm) and small acute tears do not have to be repaired, but freshening techniques should definitely be used to promote healing.

■ RAMP LESIONS (FIG. 14)

A special type of meniscal injury involves the peripheral attachment of the posterior horn of the medial meniscus and is typically associated with an ACL deficiency. It is defined as a "ramp lesion" to distinguish it from other types of posterior longitudinal tears. Ramp lesions most commonly occur in association with ACL ruptures. They may result from an acute rupture or may develop in a knee with chronic ACL deficiency. During arthroscopy, the posterior peripheral attachment of the medial meniscus should be inspected in any patient who presents with an acute or chronic ACL tear. Often, this will reveal severe lesions that would otherwise be missed and left untreated. Extension of the lesion toward the middle third could easily destabilize the entire posterior meniscus. Since resective surgery in these cases would most likely consist of a total meniscectomy, repair should always be attempted.

■ SUGGESTED READINGS

1. Karia M, Ghaly Y, Al-Hadithy N, Mordecai S, Gupte C. Current concepts in the techniques, indications and outcomes of meniscal repairs. Eur J Orthop Surg Traumatol. 2019;29(3): 509-20.
2. Strobel MJ. Manual of arthroscopic surgery. Berlin: Springer; 2002; pp. 99-199.
3. Ward BD, Lubowitz JH. Basic knee arthroscopy part 4: Chondroplasty, meniscectomy, and cruciate ligament evaluation. Arthrosc Tech. 2013;2(4):e507-8.

Posterior Cruciate Ligament

Bhushan Jaywantrao Patil, Sandeep Narayan Deore, Sachin Yashwant Kale, Pramod Bhor

ANATOMY OF THE POSTERIOR CRUCIATE LIGAMENT

The posterior cruciate ligament (PCL) is one of the four main ligaments of the knee. It is a strong, intra-articular ligament located within the intercondylar notch of the femur. Originating from the anterolateral aspect of the medial femoral condyle, the PCL inserts onto the posterior aspect of the tibial plateau, approximately 1 cm below the joint line.

The PCL is composed of two primary bundles:
1. *Anterolateral bundle (ALB)*: Tightens during knee flexion.
2. *Posteromedial bundle (PMB)*: Tightens during knee extension.

The ligament functions to resist posterior translation of the tibia relative to the femur and provides rotational stability.

CLASSIFICATION OF POSTERIOR CRUCIATE LIGAMENT INJURIES

Posterior cruciate ligament injuries are commonly classified based on their severity and mechanism:
- *Grade I*: Partial tear with mild instability.
- *Grade II*: Partial tear with moderate instability.
- *Grade III*: Complete tear with significant instability.
- *Grade IV*: PCL tear associated with injuries to other ligaments [e.g., anterior cruciate ligament (ACL), medial collateral ligament (MCL), and lateral collateral ligament (LCL)].

BIOMECHANICS OF THE POSTERIOR CRUCIATE LIGAMENT

The PCL serves as the primary restraint against posterior tibial translation, especially between 90° and 120° of knee flexion. It also contributes to medial-lateral stability and resists varus and valgus forces when combined with other ligamentous structures. The ALB and PMB work synergistically to maintain stability across different knee positions.

■ EXAMINATION FINDINGS AND CLINICAL TESTS FOR POSTERIOR CRUCIATE LIGAMENT TEARS

- *Patient history*: Often involves trauma such as a "dashboard injury" during a motor vehicle accident or a fall on a flexed knee with a plantar-flexed foot.
- *Inspection*: Swelling, posterior sag of the tibia in severe cases.
- *Palpation*: Tenderness over the posterior aspect of the knee.

Clinical Tests

- *Posterior drawer test*: With the knee flexed to 90°, posterior translation of the tibia is assessed.
- *Posterior sag sign*: Observation of posterior displacement of the tibia relative to the femur when the knee is flexed at 90°.
- *Quadriceps active test*: Dynamic test to observe anterior translation of the tibia upon quadriceps contraction.
- *Reverse pivot-shift test*: Assesses posterolateral instability associated with PCL injuries.

■ INVESTIGATIONS FOR DIAGNOSIS OF POSTERIOR CRUCIATE LIGAMENT TEARS

- *X-rays*: May reveal posterior tibial translation or avulsion fractures.
- *Stress X-rays*: Evaluate posterior laxity using posterior stress.
- *MRI*: Gold standard for assessing PCL integrity, associated injuries, and grading the severity of the tear.

Special Investigations

Arthroscopy: Provides direct visualization of PCL injuries and concurrent knee pathology **(Fig. 1)**.

Dynamic fluoroscopy: Rarely used but can assess dynamic instability during knee movement.

■ TREATMENT OF POSTERIOR CRUCIATE LIGAMENT TEARS

Nonoperative Treatment

- Indicated for grade I and II injuries or low-demand patients
- *Components*:
  - Immobilization using a posterior cruciate brace to maintain anterior tibial positioning

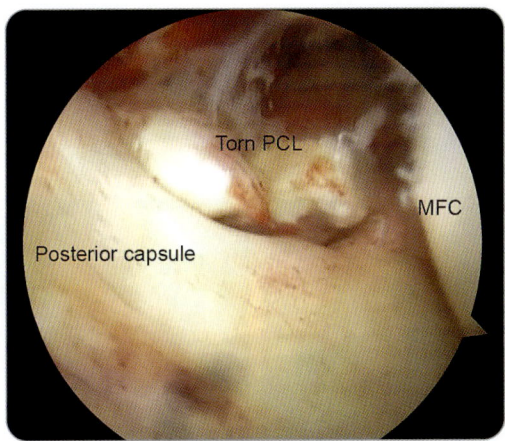

FIG. 1: Arthroscopic image showing the torn PCL.
(MFC: medial femoral condyle; PCL: posterior cruciate ligament)

- Physical therapy focused on strengthening the quadriceps
- Avoidance of activities that place posterior stress on the knee

Nonoperative Treatment: In Detail

- *Immobilization*: A posterior cruciate brace is recommended to maintain anterior tibial positioning. Typically worn for 4–6 weeks, followed by gradual weaning.
- *Physical therapy*:
  - Focus on quadriceps strengthening to compensate for posterior instability
  - Closed kinetic chain exercises to avoid stress on the PCL
  - Proprioceptive training to enhance neuromuscular control
  - Avoid hamstring activation exercises in the initial phases, as they can increase posterior tibial translation.

Outcome: Most patients with grade I and II injuries regain functional stability within 6–12 weeks.

Operative Treatment

- *Indications*: Indicated for grade III and IV injuries, avulsion fractures, or chronic instability.
- Persistent instability, combined ligament injuries, or chronic PCL deficiency leading to functional limitations.

Surgical Techniques (Figs. 2A to E)

Posterior Cruciate Ligament Reconstruction

- *Grafts used*: Autografts (bone-patellar tendon-bone, quadriceps tendon, or hamstring tendon) or allografts.

- *Single-bundle reconstruction*: Focuses on replicating the function of the ALB.
- *Double-bundle reconstruction*: Restores both anterolateral and PMB functions, providing superior biomechanical stability.

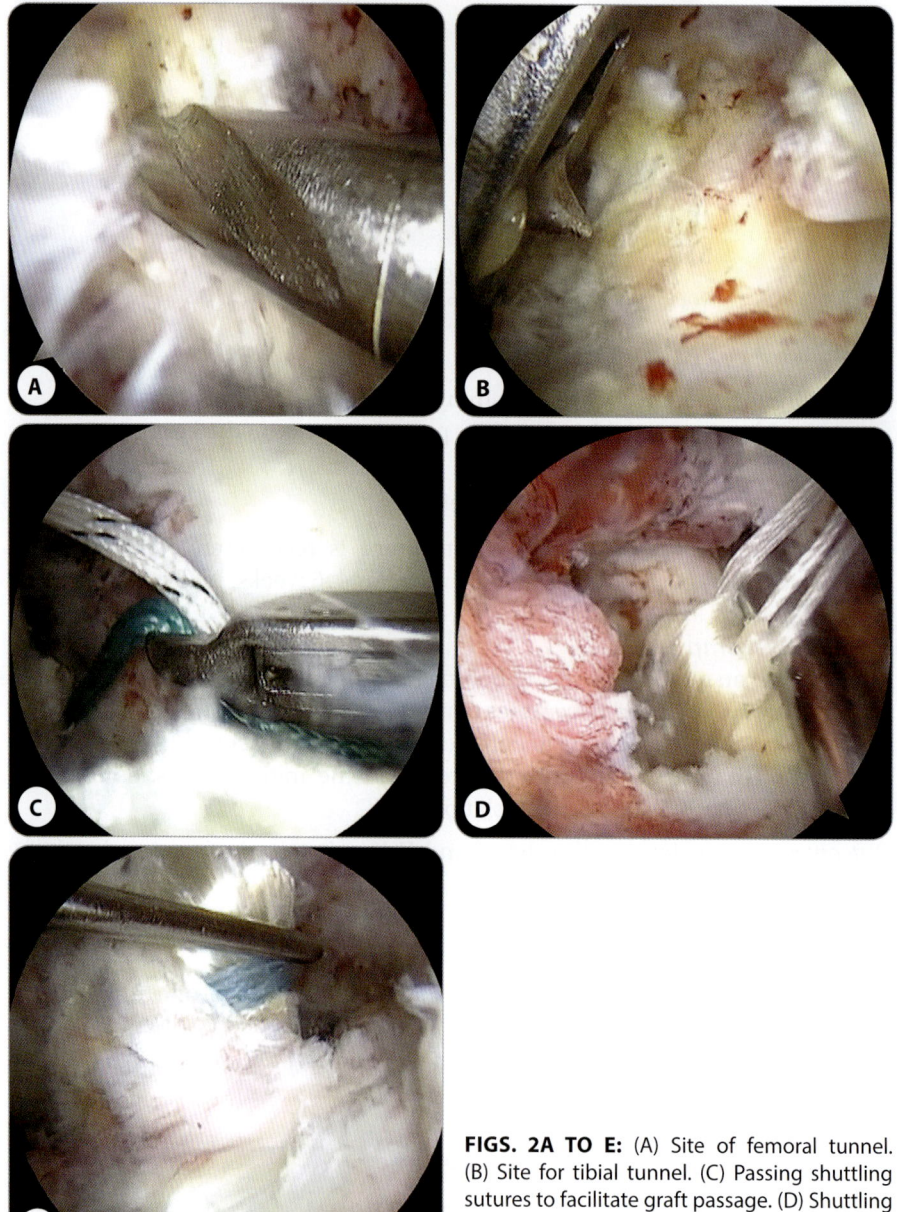

FIGS. 2A TO E: (A) Site of femoral tunnel. (B) Site for tibial tunnel. (C) Passing shuttling sutures to facilitate graft passage. (D) Shuttling the graft through the tibial tunnel. (E) PCL graft passed into the femoral tunnel.

Posterior Cruciate Ligament Repair
- Indicated for acute avulsion fractures
- Techniques include suture anchors or screw fixation of the avulsed fragment

Augmented Techniques
Augmented reconstruction involves additional fixation to enhance graft stability and prevent elongation.

NEWER METHODS OF TREATMENT FOR POSTERIOR CRUCIATE LIGAMENT INJURIES

- *Augmented PCL reconstruction*: Combines traditional grafting with additional fixation techniques for enhanced stability.
- *Biological augmentation*: Use of growth factors, stem cells, or platelet-rich plasma (PRP) to enhance healing.
- *Minimally invasive arthroscopic techniques*: Improved visualization and precision in PCL repair and reconstruction.
- *Robotics and navigation systems*: Increasing precision in graft placement and tensioning.

REVIEW OF PUBMED ARTICLES (LAST 5 YEARS)

A search on PubMed for the latest research on PCL injuries reveals the following trends:
- *Improved surgical techniques*: Studies highlight advancements in double-bundle reconstruction and fixation methods for better biomechanical outcomes.
- *Biomechanical studies*: Research emphasizes the role of anatomical reconstruction in restoring native knee kinematics.
- *Nonoperative outcomes*: Comparative studies showing effective results of nonoperative management for isolated PCL injuries.
- *Biological enhancements*: Increasing evidence supports the use of biological agents to accelerate healing and improve outcomes.
- *Long-term follow-ups*: Recent articles focus on the long-term functional and radiological outcomes of PCL reconstructions.

In conclusion, the treatment of PCL injuries has evolved significantly with the advent of advanced imaging, surgical techniques, and biological therapies. Future research is likely to focus on enhancing outcomes through personalized and minimally invasive approaches.

POSTOPERATIVE REHABILITATION

- Early controlled motion exercises within a PCL brace
- Quadriceps strengthening from the first week

- Weight-bearing restrictions until graft integration (typically 6–8 weeks)
- Return to sports in 9–12 months after achieving functional stability.

COMPLICATIONS

- Stiffness, persistent instability, and graft failure are potential risks. Regular follow-ups ensure early detection and management.
- With these expanded details and supporting visuals, the chapter aims to provide a comprehensive understanding of PCL injury management.

SUGGESTED READINGS

1. Strobel MJ. Manual of arthroscopic surgery. Berlin: Springer; 2002; pp. 571-642
2. Strobel MJ. Manual of arthroscopic surgery. Berlin: Springer; 2002.

CHAPTER 8

Shoulder Positioning, Draping, and Portals

Pramod Bhor, Rahul V Davari, Sachin Yashwant Kale, Rohit Mahesh Sane

■ POSITIONING

Two positioning methods are commonly used for shoulder arthroscopy: (1) the lateral decubitus position and (2) the beach chair position. Each has its own advantages and disadvantages.

Lateral Decubitus Position (Figs. 1A and B)

The patient is placed in a lateral position with the back even with the edge of the table. The torso is supported by side rests mounted anteriorly at the level of the thoracic outlet and posteriorly at the level of the pelvis. Bony prominences (elbow and fibular head on the downside) are carefully padded.

It should be considered that the glenoid cavity of the scapula serves as the reference plane for the glenohumeral joint. If the patient is positioned in strict lateral decubitus, the articular surface of the glenohumeral joint will be tilted anteriorly. This joint is directed laterally either by rolling back the patient's torso about 30° onto a beanbag or by tilting the operating table.

This position requires a special shoulder traction system that permits adjustments in abduction, anteversion, and distraction. A forearm wrap connects the arm securely to an overhead traction device without risk of localized compression injury to the soft tissues. The arm is positioned in approximately 45° of abduction and 15° of anteversion with a traction weight of 4–8 kg. More than 45° of abduction or heavier traction could lead to brachial plexus injury.

Advantages
- Free access to the scapula
- Controlled amount of arm traction
- Facilitates glenohumeral surgery

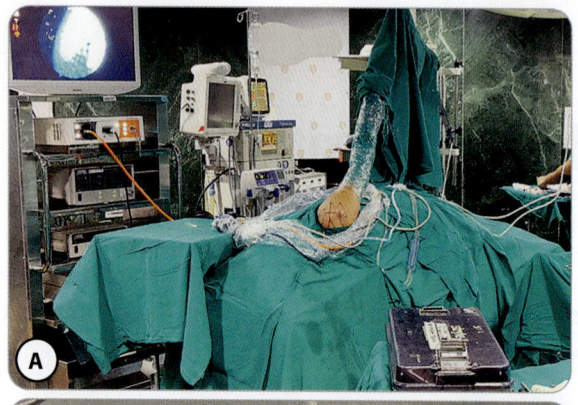
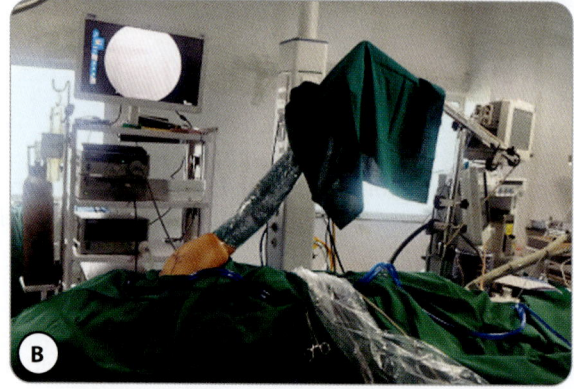

FIGS. 1A AND B: Final setup in lateral position.

Disadvantages

The disadvantages are need for traction device (arm holder), time consuming, greater risk of position-related injuries (localized pressure injury to the down arm, plexus stretch injury), complex padding, complex draping, and difficult conversion to an open procedure.

Beach Chair Position

When this position is used, it is important to keep the full circumference of the shoulder accessible during the operation. An extended head rest is used that supports the head and places the shoulder past the edge of the operating table so that it is accessible from both the anterior and posterior sides **(Fig. 2)**.

Advantages

- Allows for rapid conversion to an open procedure
- Normal vertical orientation of shoulder anatomy
- Well suited for subacromial procedures
- Lower cost

CHAPTER 8: Shoulder Positioning, Draping, and Portals   77

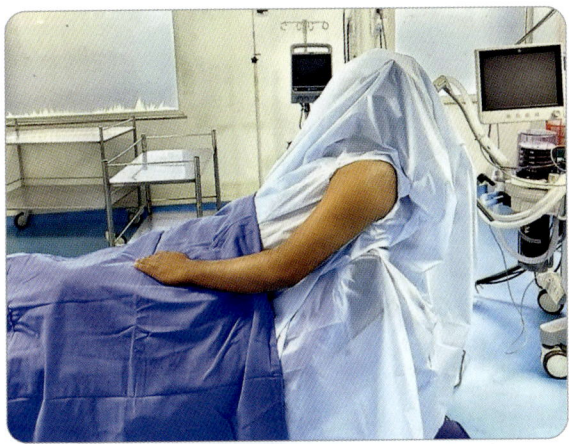

FIG. 2: Beach chair position.

- Saves time and facilitates draping
- Easier conversion to open surgery

Disadvantages
- Difficult or poor visualization of the medial scapular margin
- Risk of hypotensive brain injury

■ DRAPING

Draping technique depends on the position.

Lateral Decubitus Position

For arthroscopy in the lateral decubitus position, the patient should be covered with a drape prior to skin preparation to protect the patient from antiseptic solution running off the skin. The arm is sterilely wrapped and secured in the traction device, and the shoulder area is covered with two sterile aperture drapes, one placed from the axillary side and the other from the cranial side **(Fig. 3)**.

Beach Chair Position

For beach chair arthroscopy, the arm is abducted at the shoulder during the skin preparation; a towel protects the patient's body from solution running off the skin. Next, the patient is covered to the chest with sterile fabric drapes. A waterproof adhesive aperture sheet is placed over the shoulder from the cranial side, and a smaller adhesive drape is placed from the axillary side. The arm is wrapped in a waterproof towel drape secured with adhesive tape. The cranial sheet is stretched over the patient's head to form a screen for the anesthesiologist, who sits next to the contralateral shoulder.

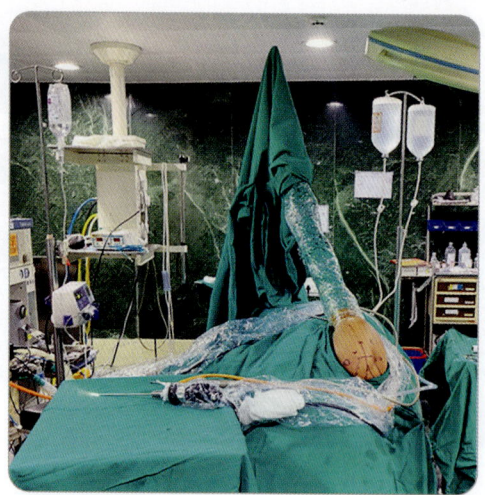

FIG. 3: Final draping for lateral position.

◼ PORTALS (FIG. 4)

When the beach chair position is used, the surgeon stands posterolateral to the operative shoulder. This area is not accessible to the anesthesiologist, who sits cranial to the contralateral shoulder. The first assistant stands lateral to the patient's upper arm, and the scrub nurse stands next to the instrument table at the level of the patient's pelvis. The arthroscopy cart is on the opposite side of the operating table.

Before the portals are created, it is necessary to palpate the bony structures about the shoulder. The principal landmarks are the clavicle, acromioclavicular (AC) joint, acromion, coracoid process, and scapular spine.

The entire shoulder is covered by the deltoid muscle. The anterior portion of the muscle arises from the lateral half of the clavicle, its middle portion from the acromion, and its posterior portion from the scapular spine. It inserts on the deltoid tuberosity of the humerus. The anterior, lateral, and posterior portals penetrate the deltoid muscle, and its fibers can be seen as the arthroscope is withdrawn at the end of the procedure.

The axillary nerve supplies the deltoid muscle and passes with the posterior circumflex humeral artery through the axillary quadrangular space, which is bounded above by the inferior border of the teres minor muscle. Thus, the axillary nerve relates closely to the "classic" posterior portal for glenohumeral arthroscopy.

Glenohumeral Portals (Figs. 4 and 5)

Posterior Portal

This portal serves as the primary visualization portal. It is placed approximately 2–3 cm inferior and 1–2 cm medial to the posterolateral corner of the

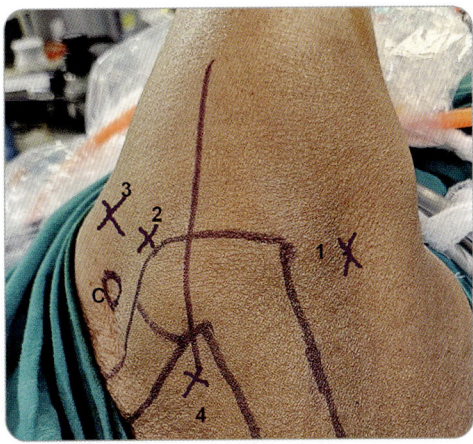

FIG. 4: Image showing all common portals for shoulder arthroscopy, 1—posterior, 2—anterior–superior, 3—anterior–inferior, 4—Neviaser portal, and C—coracoid process.

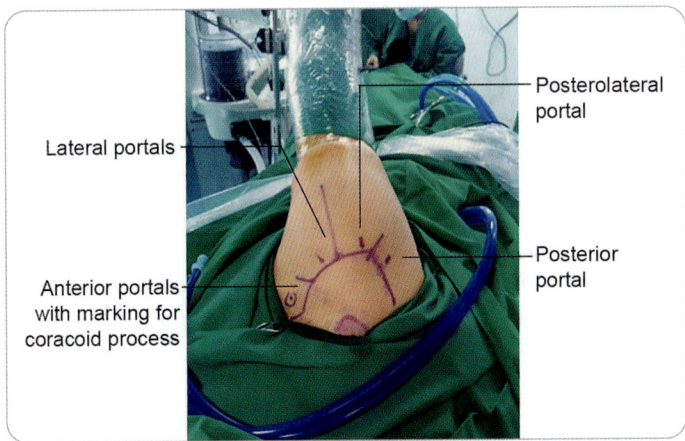

FIG. 5: Image showing all common portals for shoulder arthroscopy.

acromion. This position corresponds to the palpable "soft spot" of the posterior shoulder.

Anterior Portals

The two anterior portals: Anterior–superior and anterior–inferior—are used for instrumentation or inflow. They can also be used to inspect the posterior portion of the glenohumeral joint after the arthroscope and instrument portals have been switched.

Anterior-Superior portal: This portal is established just anterior to the biceps tendon. This is the main viewing portal for labral surgery. With the scope in this portal, a bird's eye view of the glenoid is seen.

Anterior-Inferior portal: This portal is placed just proximal to the subscapularis tendon at the apex of the rotator interval. This is the working portal while doing a Bankart repair. Structures most at risk from the anterior portals are the cephalic vein in the deltopectoral interval and the musculocutaneous nerve. The latter runs about 4–5 cm inferior to the coracoid process but may be as close as 1 cm to the coracoid process if it perforates the coracobrachialis muscle at that level.

Superior Portal

The superior portal (Neviaser portal, supraspinatus portal) is placed approximately 1 cm medial to the acromion between the clavicle and scapular spine and is used for instrumentation or inflow. Structures at risk are the suprascapular nerve and suprascapular artery, which run in the scapular notch. The scapular notch is located about 2 cm medial to this portal.

Subacromial Portals (Fig. 4)

Subacromial arthroscopy is possible through posterior, anterior, lateral, and superior portals.

Posterior Subacromial Portal

The same skin incision is used as for the posterior glenohumeral portal. Creation of the portal is facilitated by placing it just 1–1.5 cm inferior to the posterolateral corner of the acromion.

Anterior Subacromial Portal

This portal is placed lateral to the coracoacromial ligament.

Lateral Subacromial Portal

This portal is placed distal to the lateral acromial border under arthroscopic vision. It is located approximately 2 cm posterior to the anterolateral acromion and just below the subacromial sulcus, which is usually palpable. The portal should take the shortest path through the soft tissues into the subacromial space to facilitate outflow and avoid excessive fluid collection in the subcutaneous tissue.

Superior Subacromial Portal

The subacromial space can also be reached from the superior glenohumeral portal.

Acromioclavicular Portals

An anterior and a posterosuperior portal are known. Both give direct access to the AC joint. Alternatively, the AC joint can be reached through the subacromial space.

Creating the Glenohumeral Posterior Viewing Portal: Technique

The portal is created in the following sequence of steps.

Palpation

The soft spot between the infraspinatus and teres minor muscles is palpated approximately 1–2 cm inferior and 1 cm medial to the posterolateral corner of the acromion.

Skin Incision

A 3–4-mm incision is made through the skin only. A deeper incision is avoided, as it could needlessly transect deltoid muscle fibers and cause bleeding.

Sheath Insertion

The sheath with blunt obturator is advanced toward the glenohumeral joint and coracoid process with a careful twisting motion. As the sheath is twisted during insertion, the obturator will penetrate the deltoid bluntly by pushing its fibers aside. The tip of the blunt obturator is used to palpate the posterior glenoid rim and humeral head and locate the intervening joint space. The capsule is penetrated on the joint line. A marked decrease in resistance confirms that the sheath has entered the glenohumeral joint.

Distention

The joint is distended with fluid. To make certain that the fluid is distending the glenohumeral joint rather than extra-articular soft tissues, the blunt obturator is removed and the scope inserted. If intra-articular structures can be seen after several milliliters of fluid have been instilled, the distention is continued. If articular structures (humeral head or biceps tendon) cannot be seen, the sheath may be outside the joint.

Creating the Glenohumeral Instrument Portal: Technique (Figs. 6 to 14)

Either of two techniques can be used to create the anterior instrument portals:
1. *Inside-out technique using a switching stick (Wissinger rod)*: The scope with sheath is placed in close contact with the rotator interval. Keeping the sheath in place, the scope is removed. The Wissinger rod is then passed in the sheath and pushed through the rotator interval till it is impinging on the skin. A stab incision is then taken over the tip of the Wissinger rod and the rod is then pulled out of the incision. The sheath is withdrawn back into the joint keeping the other tip of the Wissinger rod into the joint. A scope is reinserted into the sheath and dilator and cannula is placed over the Wissinger rod in the anteroinferior portal.

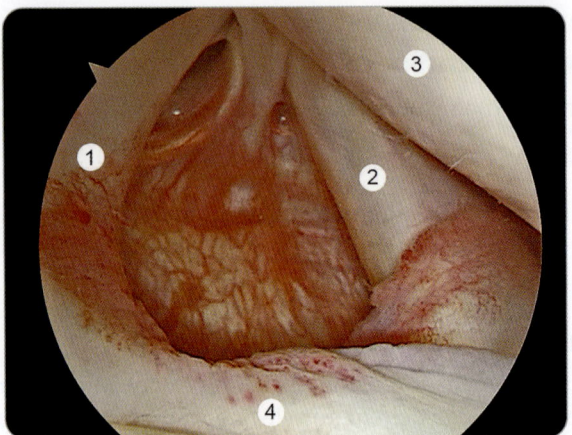

FIG. 6: Intra-articular arthroscopic view of the shoulder, 1—long head of biceps (LHB), 2—subscapularis, 3—humeral head, 4—anterior labrum.

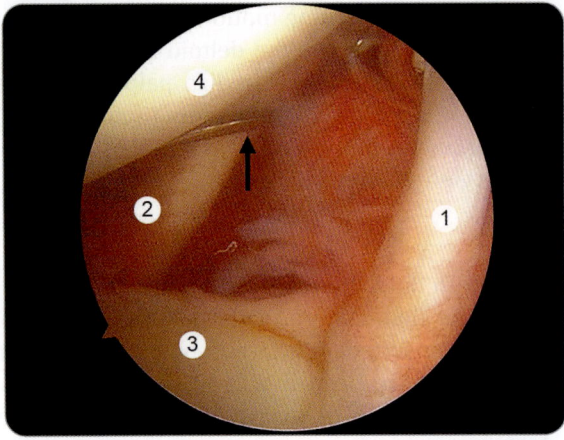

FIG. 7: Arrow—needle, 1—long head of biceps (LHB), 2—subscapularis, 3—glenoid, 4—humeral head.

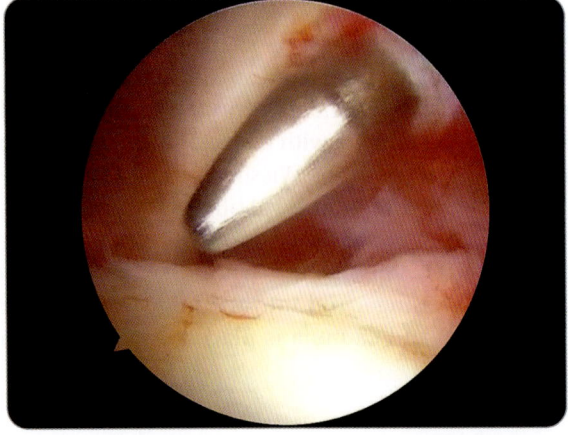

FIG. 8: Anterior portal entry with stiching rod.

CHAPTER 8: Shoulder Positioning, Draping, and Portals

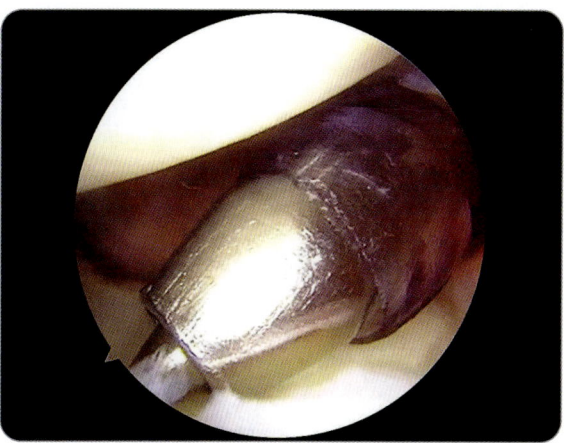

FIG. 9: Entry with dilator with 8 mm canola.

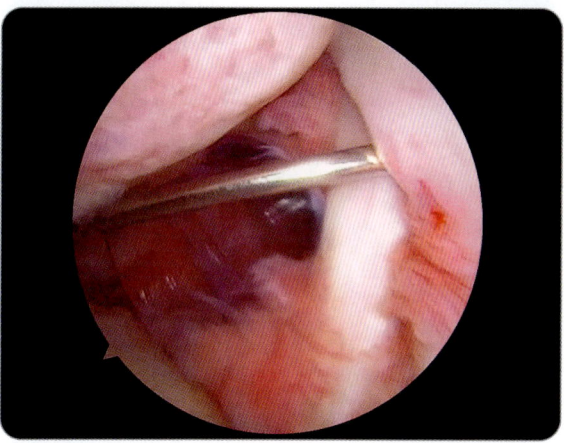

FIG. 10: Making entry with a needle in the anterosuperior (AS) portal.

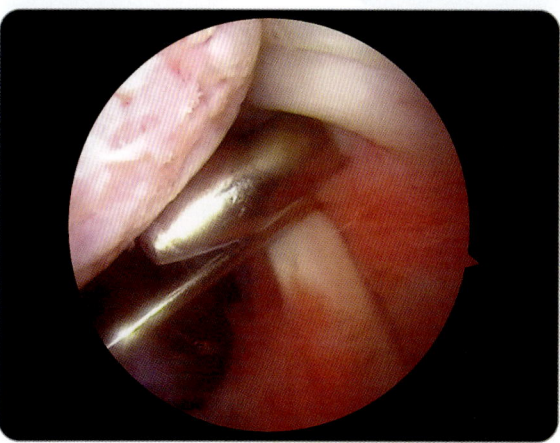

FIG. 11: Stitching rod through anterosuperior (AS) portal.

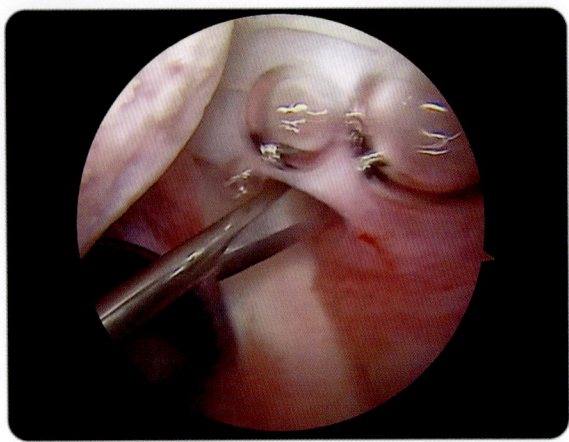

FIG. 12: Making entry with a blade and port in the anterosuperior (AS).

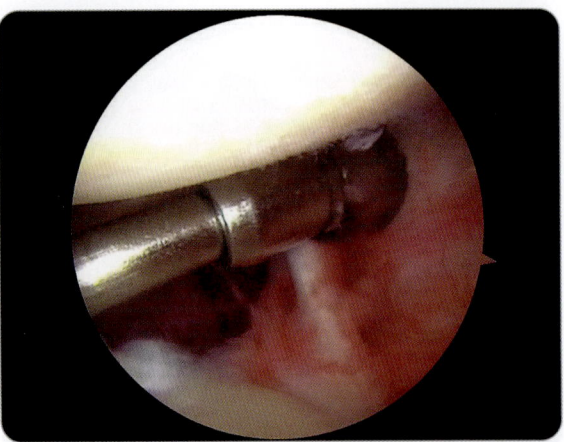

FIG. 13: Entry with 5 mm canola in anterosuperior (AS).

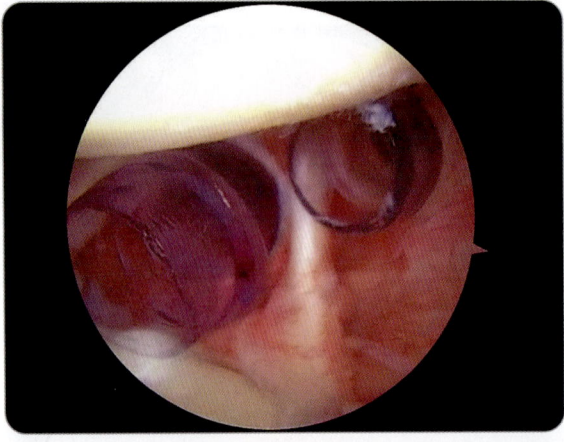

FIG. 14: Final anterior–superior and anterior-inferior portals.

2. *Outside-in technique using a percutaneous needle*: An 18-G spinal needle is used placed percutaneously into the joint under vision. A stab incision is taken along the needle up to the capsule. A Wissinger rod is placed along the needle into the joint. Needle is then removed and a dilator and cannula is placed.

Creating the Subacromial Arthroscope Portal: Technique (Fig. 15)

This portal is created following arthroscopic inspection of the glenohumeral joint.

Positioning the Patient

When arthroscopy is performed in the lateral decubitus position, it may be necessary to decrease arm abduction to 15° and rotate the arm slightly forward while keeping it extended. Initially the arthroscope remains in the glenohumeral joint. The scope is then withdrawn, and a blunt obturator is inserted into the sheath.

Entering the Subacromial Space

The sheath with obturator inserted is backed out of the glenohumeral joint. The sheath can be felt exiting the joint space. The obturator-armed sheath is then angled superiorly and advanced toward the acromion. It is first swept medially and laterally to lyse bursal adhesions that would obstruct vision.

Improving Orientation

Percutaneous needles can be inserted at the lateral border and anterolateral corner of the acromion and at the AC joint to improve orientation in the subacromial space after insertion of the scope.

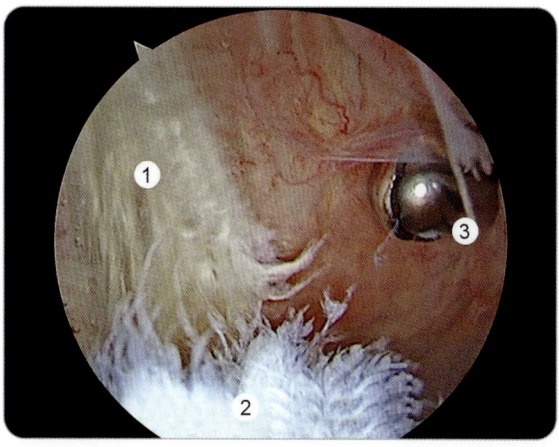

FIG. 15: Subacromial view from the posterior portal, showing 1—contact lesion on CA ligament, 2—subacromial bursa, and 3—instrumental portal with shaver.

Creating the Subacromial Instrument Portal: Technique

An anterior instrument portal is created next. This can be done from inside-out using a Wissinger rod or switching stick, as described for the glenohumeral joint, or from outside-in using a percutaneous needle.

This superficial joint can be entered with a percutaneous needle from the anterior side and distended with fluid. The arthroscope portal is created by inserting a second needle from the posterosuperior side. Fluid backflow confirms that the needle is intra-articular. A 1-2-mm skin incision is made at the insertion site, the subcutaneous tissue is carefully spread open, and a sheath with blunt obturator is inserted. Because the AC joint is very small, we recommend using the "wrist scope" from the small joint instrument set. The anterior needle remains in the AC joint and, if necessary, can be used to redistend the joint.

When the sheath is within the joint and the scope has been inserted, the inflow line is connected to the sheath. The needle technique is used to establish the anterior portal, which is used for instrumentation (e.g., motorized instruments for resecting the articular disk or the lateral end of the clavicle).

■ SUGGESTED READING

1. Strobel MJ. Manual of arthroscopic surgery. Berlin: Springer; 2002. pp. 876-84.

CHAPTER 9

Diagnostic Round (Shoulder), Indications and Complications

Prasad Liladhar Chaudhari, Rohit Mahesh Sane, Sandeep Narayan Deore, Sachin Yashwant Kale

■ EXAMINATION OF THE GLENOHUMERAL JOINT

After the arthroscope has been inserted into the joint and carefully retracted, the first structures to be identified are usually the glenoid and the anterior part of the labrum.

Angling the arthroscope upward brings the long biceps tendon into view **(Fig. 1)**. This tendon is the most important primary landmark for intra-articular orientation. Its entire course can be seen, including its origin on the supraglenoid tubercle and labrum. The biceps tendon runs forward over the humeral head and enters the bicipital groove **(Fig. 2)**.

Next the anterior capsule and the anterior part of the glenoid and labrum are evaluated. An important landmark on the anterior capsule is the triangle between the subscapularis tendon, superior glenohumeral ligament, and middle glenohumeral ligament. The free edge of the subscapularis tendon is easily

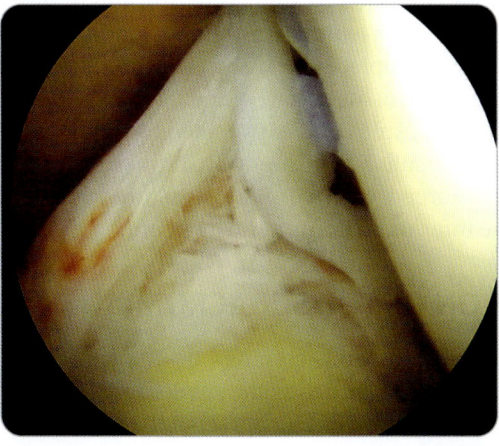

FIG.1: Intra-articular view of the glenohumeral joint showing long head of the biceps (LHB) anchor and lesion, and labral pathology.

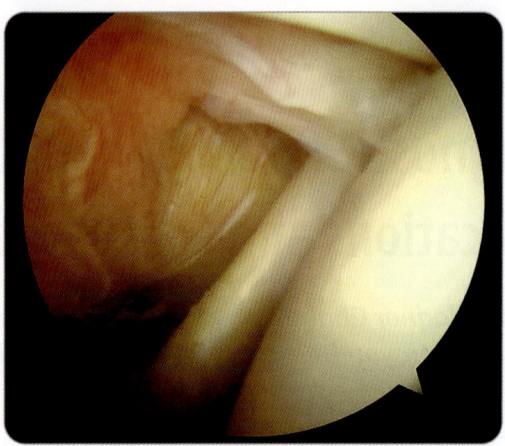

FIG. 2: Intra-articular view of the glenohumeral joint showing long head of the biceps (LHB) around the groove and subscapularis in front.

identified in most cases. It is an important landmark for placing the anterior inferior portal.

The anterior portion of the labrum is inspected. It can display many possible anatomic variants in addition to pathologic separations [superior labral anterior to posterior (SLAP) lesions and Andrews lesion].

Distal to the middle glenohumeral ligament, the inferior glenohumeral ligament runs almost parallel to the glenoid. It usually appears as a bandlike thickening of the capsule that opens distally toward the inferior recess.

The arthroscope can be retracted to evaluate the glenoid and the posterior glenoid rim as far as the inferior recess. Angling the scope downward demonstrates the inferior part of the labrum and, below it, the axillary recess.

From there the arthroscope is swung back upward along the humeral head. The posterior aspect of the humeral head features the "bare spot" which should not be mistaken for a Hill–Sachs lesion. The insertion of the rotator tendons on the greater tuberosity (supra- and infraspinatus tendons) can be identified and inspected for partial or complete tears. The arm should be abducted at this time to better visualize the area of insertion.

The posterior joint capsule can be inspected by moving the arthroscope to an anterior portal. The capsule is considerably thinner posteriorly than anteriorly. Sometimes it is reinforced by a cordlike structure representing the posterior inferior band of the inferior glenohumeral ligament.

■ EXAMINATION OF THE SUBACROMIAL SPACE

First the sheath with blunt obturator has been swept back-and-forth to lyse fibrous bands and adhesions, and then the subacromial space is distended. At this point, the extent of the space can be appreciated. Some anatomic structures are usually difficult or impossible to identify because they are covered by synovium. When a partial synovectomy is performed, the rotator cuff on the floor of the subacromial space can be identified and evaluated for pathology. The acromion and coracoacromial ligament can be identified in the superior portion of the space.

INDICATIONS

- Chronic pain
- Locking
- Loose bodies
- Labral lesions
- Rotator cuff tears
- Subacromial syndrome
- Restricted range of motion (ROM)
- Biceps lesions
- Shoulder instability
- Infection
- Acromioclavicular (AC) joint arthropathies

COMPLICATIONS

Complication rates of 0.8–3% have been reported for shoulder arthroscopy. As in other joints, there is probably a high unreported incidence of iatrogenic cartilage lesions. It should be stressed, however, that fluid extravasation occurs in almost every arthroscopic shoulder operation and is not considered a complication. Even pronounced extravasation will generally resolve in 1–2 hours without sequelae. It may interfere with the surgical procedure, however, by making it difficult to insert operating instruments. Obscured vision due to bleeding is another very frequent problem in arthroscopic operations.

The following types of complications are discussed here.

Position-related Complications

The beach chair position is associated with postural hypotension, and the anesthesiologist must be prepared for this. Hypoglossal nerve injury has also been reported with this position; it can be prevented by adequate padding.

The lateral decubitus position may be associated with pressure injury to the ulnar nerve in the arm and peroneal nerve in the leg on the downside. Careful padding is necessary.

Distraction-related Complications

More than 8 kg of traction places strain on the brachial plexus and may even cause traction injury. The traction weight should not exceed 8 kg, therefore. Also, the arm should not be abducted by >45°. Traction injuries to the musculocutaneous nerve have been described. The hand and forearm should be carefully padded and adequately secured to the traction device to avoid local pressure injuries and skin lesions.

Portal-related Complications

A faulty insertion angle can cause undesired entry of the sheath into the subdeltoid bursa or axilla.

Cartilage Lesions

Forcible or aggressive sheath insertion can cause scuffing or scraping injuries to the articular cartilage on the humeral head or glenoid. Labral lesions can also occur.

Nerve Lesions

- *Axillary nerve*: Placing the posterior glenohumeral portal 3–5 cm inferior to the acromion poses a risk to the axillary nerve. Since the nerve is also very close to the axillary recess, it may be injured by an aggressive synovectomy or capsular incisions in the lower part of the joint.
- *Suprascapular nerve*: This nerve runs an average of 1.8 cm medial to the glenohumeral joint. It runs about 3 cm medial to the superior glenohumeral portal.
- *Infraspinous branch of the suprascapular nerve*: This nerve branch is at risk during repairs of the anterior capsule and ligaments and transglenoidal fixation.
- *Brachial plexus*: The brachial plexus or its branches (median nerve, ulnar nerve, and musculocutaneous nerve) are at risk during placement of the anterior portals. As a result, the inside-out Wissinger rod technique is often used in establishing the anterior inferior glenohumeral portal.
- *Musculocutaneous nerve*: This nerve arises from the lateral part of the brachial plexus and runs 2.5–4 cm distal to the tip of the coracoid process. It can penetrate the coracobrachialis muscle at varying levels, and sometimes it runs just 1 cm inferior to the coracoid process. Consequently, the anterior portals should not be placed distal and medial to the tip of the coracoid process.

Technique-related Complications

Instrument Breakage

Instrument breakage is a danger in shoulder arthroscopy as in any other arthroscopic procedure. It can be very difficult to locate instrument fragments that have slipped into the variable recesses of the glenohumeral joint.

Nerve Lesions

Nerves that run anterior or posterior to the glenoid (e.g., the suprascapular nerve and infrascapular branch) are at risk during repairs of the anterior capsule and ligaments.

Loosening or Breakage of Fixation Hardware

Staple fixation was commonly used in the early days of arthroscopic shoulder stabilization. It was not unusual for the staples to loosen or break out of the bone. As a result, staple fixation is no longer practiced today.

Bony Lesions

A bone fragment may be broken from the glenoid during the fixation of anterior labral structures.

Rotator Cuff Tears

Aggressive debridement can convert a partial rotator cuff tear to a full-thickness tear. Partial cuff tears should be debrided with extreme care, therefore.

Acromial Fracture

Excessive resection during subacromial decompression can greatly thin the acromion, predisposing it to fracture by even minor trauma. Thus, before performing subacromial decompression the surgeon should evaluate the thickness of the acromion, which is highly variable.

Clavicular Fracture

Part of the inferior clavicle is often removed during subacromial decompression. Excessive resection in this area can predispose to clavicular fracture.

Infection

Without doubt, infection is the most feared complication of shoulder arthroscopy.

Postoperative Hemarthrosis

This complication may follow an extensive synovectomy.

■ SUGGESTED READING

1. Strobel MJ (Ed). Manual of Arthroscopic Surgery. Berlin: Springer; 2002. pp. 886-94.

CHAPTER 10

Rotator Cuff

Sandeep Narayan Deore, Pramod Bhor, Sunil H Shetty, Sachin Yashwant Kale

ANATOMY OF ROTATOR CUFF

The tendons of the subscapularis, supraspinatus, infraspinatus, and teres minor muscles form the functionally important complex of the rotator cuff. The infraspinatus muscle arises in the infraspinous fossa and inserts on the posterior facet of the greater tuberosity of the humerus. The teres minor muscle runs just inferior to the infraspinatus **(Fig. 1)**.

The supraspinatus muscle arises in the supraspinous fossa and inserts on the middle facet of the greater tuberosity. The subscapularis muscle, which arises in the subscapular fossa and inserts on the lesser tuberosity, completes the rotator cuff. Newer studies have shown that these tendons unite near rotator cable, interdigitate and merge with the capsule before inserting on the common footprint of greater tuberosity.

Rotator cuff has a depressor effect on humeral head against which deltoid functions as abductor of shoulder joint.

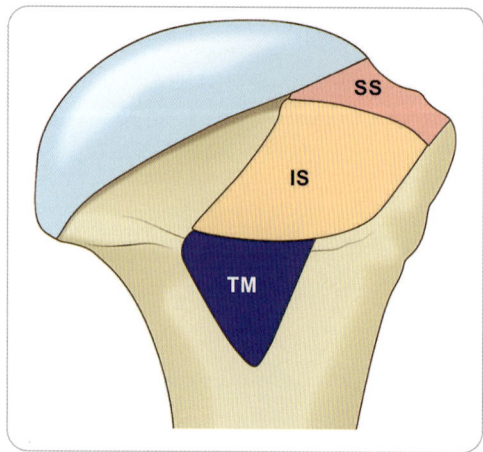

FIG. 1: Insertion of the rotator cuff on the greater tuberosity.
(IS: infraspinatus; SS: supraspinatus; TM: teres minor)

The rotator cuff forms the roof of the glenohumeral joint and the floor of the subacromial space. Thus, an intact rotator cuff prevents entry into the subacromial space from the glenohumeral joint.

■ ETIOLOGY OF ROTATOR CUFF TEAR

Rotator cuff lesions are among the most common shoulder lesions. Traumatic tears are rare except in cases of massive shoulder trauma. Most rotator cuff tears result from extensive degenerative changes based on the very high stresses that act on the cuff and other adverse mechanical factors. The most important of these factors is the very confined space beneath the acromion, due in part to the coracoacromial ligament stretching between the coracoid process and the acromion. This situation predisposes to early degenerative cuff changes, and histologic signs of tendon degeneration can be found in most individuals over 30 years of age. The relatively poor blood supply to the rotator cuff serves to exacerbate this "natural" attrition process.

On imaging studies, greater acromion index, greater critical shoulder angle (≥ 35), and smaller glenoid version angle were identified factors associated with symptomatic rotator cuff tear.

Mechanically, the tendon degeneration leads to surface irregularities and fraying. Degenerative tears usually start on the undersurface of the rotator cuff near the greater tuberosity. This type of tear, which is located on glenohumeral side is called an articular side tear (type A tear). Tears on the superior surface of the rotator cuff are known as bursal side tears (type B tears).

The degenerative surface irregularities on the rotator cuff interfere with tendon gliding and promote irritation of the subacromial space (subacromial bursitis).

These changes most commonly affect individuals who do strenuous manual work, especially when it involves repetitive overhead lifting or prolonged periods of abduction (e.g., painters and hairdressers). Various types of sport (e.g., tennis, squash, volleyball, and weightlifting) can also predispose to degenerative cuff changes.

■ CLINICAL FEATURES (FIGS. 2 TO 7)

There is history of gradual progression of shoulder pain of degenerative tendon disease. Patients give history of minor traumatic events that lead to an exacerbation of preexisting complaints.

Patients typically describe arm pain during movements of forward flexion and abduction. They also complain of nocturnal pain which aggravates in supine position and partially relieved on sitting up. Patients also experience significant weakness or "pseudoparalysis" in abduction and external rotation.

Patients above 60 years of age present with these symptoms on trivial trauma like lifting a bucket of water and household fall on outstretched hand. Younger patients have history of high velocity trauma such as contact sports and calisthenic activities.

Some patients typically claim to have felt a pop in the shoulder accompanied by severe pain.

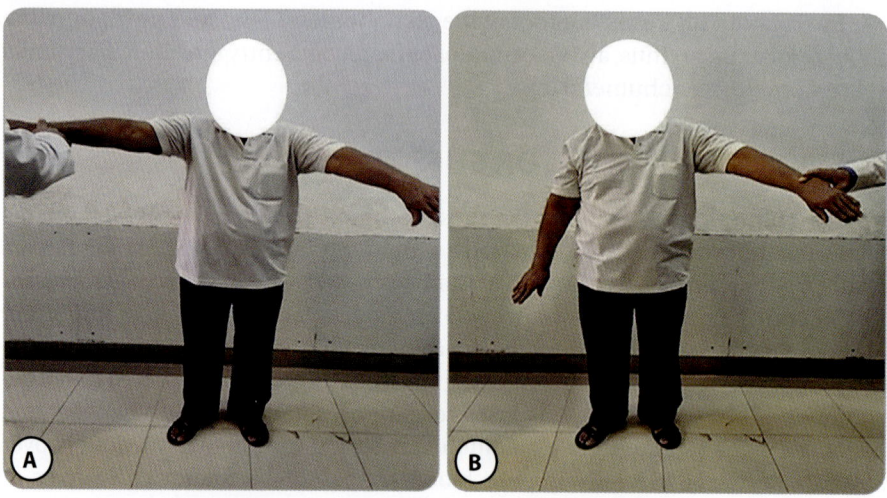

FIGS. 2A AND B: Jobe test: Weakness in forward flexion in scapular plane.

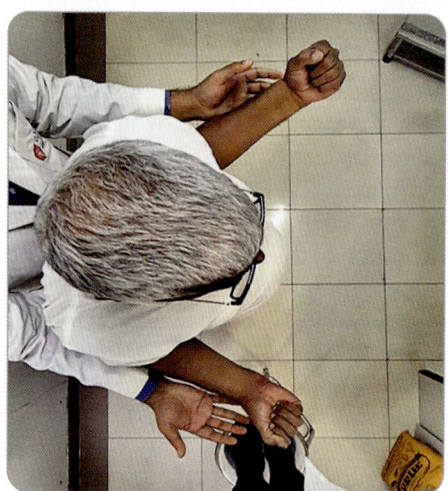

FIG. 3: Weakness in external rotation, ER lag sign.

It should also be noted that shoulder dislocations in patients over 40 years of age are frequently associated with a rotator cuff tear. In fact, in many cases, it is primary cause of shoulder dislocation than the conventional Bankart lesion as found during the surgery.

With a partial-thickness tear, marked tenderness is noted over the greater tuberosity at the insertion of the supraspinatus muscle. This is accompanied by a painful arc and a positive Jobe test.

Surprisingly many patients with massive tears present without pseudoparalysis. The cause for this may be balanced force couples on anterior (subscapularis) and posterior (teres minor) side of the joint. If either of these are torn, patients present with pseudoparalysis.

On palpation, there is tenderness over the greater tuberosity accompanied by crepitus on passive rotation of the upper arm. There can be variable atrophy of the supraspinatus and infraspinatus region.

Drop-arm sign: Weakness in abduction in the arc of 60–120°.
Hornblower sign.
Weakness in external rotation, external lag (ER) sign **(Fig. 3)**.

*Tests for subscapularis **(Fig 4)***: Gerber's lift off test.

Belly press test: Refer to **Figure 5**

Bear hug test: Refer to **Figure 6**

Speed test: Refer to **Figure 7**

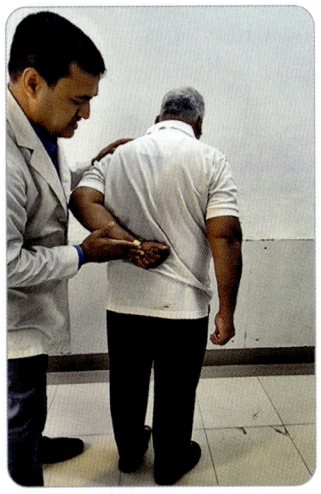

FIG. 4: Lift off test.

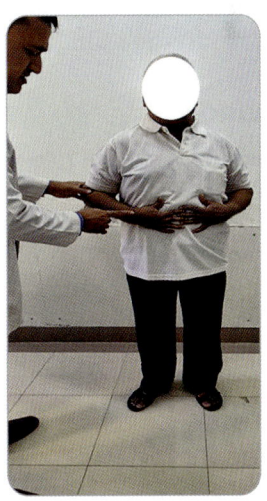

FIG. 5: Belly press test.

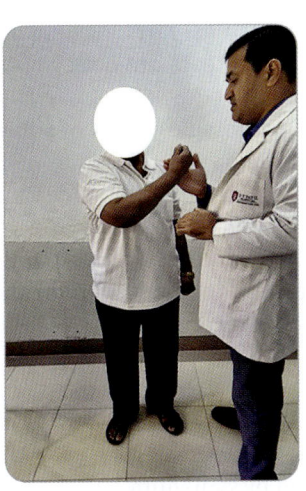

FIG. 6: Bear hug test.

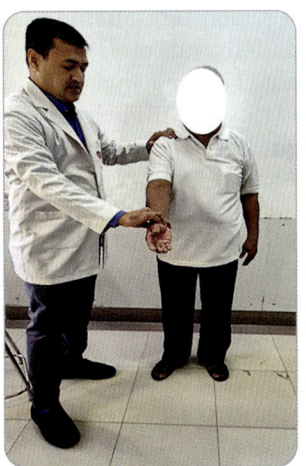

FIG. 7: Speed test.

RADIOGRAPHS

Radiographs may demonstrate sclerotic or lytic areas in the greater tuberosity, subacromial spur is a frequent finding in patients with rotator cuff tear. A chronic retracted full-thickness tear is often associated with superior migration of the humeral head with reduced acromiohumeral distance (AHD). Associated degenerative changes such as acromioclavicular joint arthropathy and glenohumeral osteophytes are also present.

The AHD is determined on the anteroposterior view with the arm in the neutral position. The normal distance is between 7 and 14 mm. The critical value is 7 mm; a distance <7 mm implies that rotator cuff repair will not yield a favorable result. Thus, the radiographic AHD is a very useful index for predicting the efficacy of a rotator cuff repair.

Calcific tendinitis which also presents with shoulder pain may show opacities near tendon insertion which can be missed on MRI images.

Ultrasound

Ultrasound has a special role in evaluating the rotator cuff and acromial bursa. The deltoid muscle and humeral head contour can also be evaluated. The sensitivity of ultrasound in the diagnosis of full-thickness rotator cuff tears is 97%, which is equivalent to that of contrast arthrography. Because ultrasound can also define structural changes, it is superior to any other technique for detecting partial-thickness tears, especially intratendinous tears located on the bursal side. This capability makes ultrasound the modality of first choice in the diagnosis of rotator cuff lesions.

Magnetic Resonance Imaging

The condition of the rotator cuff can also be evaluated with MRI. *Coronal images* help to quantify the medial retraction of the torn tendon, associated superior labral anterior posterior (SLAP) tears and thickening of inferior glenohumeral capsular pouch **(Figs. 8 and 9)**. Partial tears such as partial articular supraspinatus tendon avulsion (PASTA) and bursal-sided tears are better visualized on T2-weighted coronal images.

Axial cuts on MRI help to identify labral pathologies, tears of subscapularis, teres minor, and biceps tendon displacement **(Figs. 8 and 9)**.

Sagittal cuts on MRI help to classify tear in sagittal plane such as anterosuperior, superior or posterior quadrant. Also sagittal cuts show the amount of fatty degeneration and wasting of rotator cuff around scapular spine helping the surgeon to predict the success of rotator cuff repair surgery or the need of advanced procedures such as superior capsular reconstruction (SCR) or tendon transfer procedures.

ARTHROSCOPIC FINDINGS

The normal rotator cuff is smooth and covered by synovium.

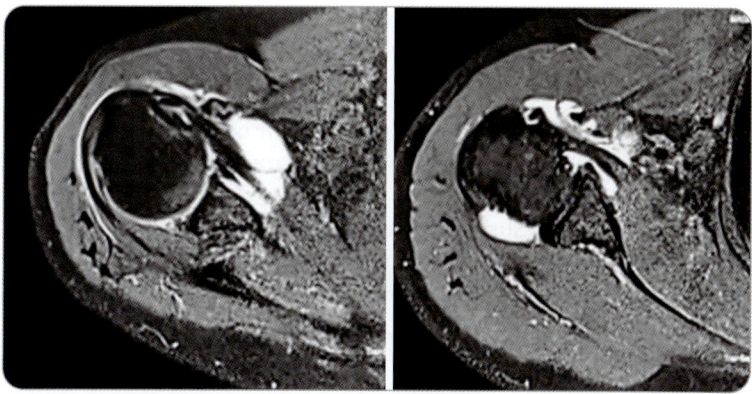

FIG. 8: Axial magnetic resonance imaging (MRI) images.

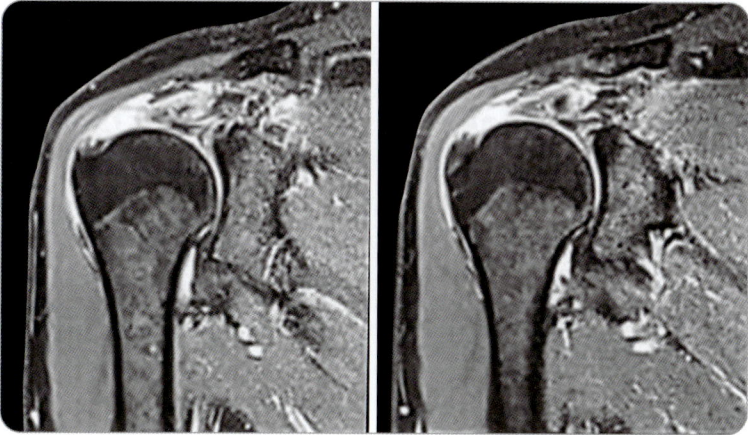

FIG. 9: Coronal magnetic resonance imaging (MRI) images.

■ PARTIAL TEAR

Degenerative partial-thickness rotator cuff tears usually start at the insertion of the cuff on the greater tuberosity, where degenerative fraying can be found. In later stages, numerous fibers become separated and present the features of an articular side partial tear (type A tear). Palpation with the probe is necessary to determine whether the tear is partial or full thickness. Most partial-thickness tears occur in zone B. Endoscopy of the subacromial space can demonstrate bursal side (type B) tears.

Tear Classification

With a complete rotator cuff tear, the subacromial space can be visualized from the glenohumeral joint. The quality of the torn tendon edge is evaluated arthroscopically, as this will have a bearing on the operative procedure. With an acute, usually traumatic cuff tear, the tear margin is covered with blood. If the tendon edge is thinned, has a soft consistency, or is indurated or even atrophic, repair will be technically more difficult. The location of the tear is also assessed.

Tear localization is aided by subdividing the rotator cuff into zones:
- *Zone A*: Anterior zone (subscapularis tendon, rotator interval, and long biceps tendon)
- *Zone B*: Superior zone (supraspinatus tendon)
- *Zone C*: Posterior zone (infraspinatus and teres minor tendons)
A line drawn along the axis of the scapular spine separates zones B and C.

The size of the tear (greatest width of the defect) is defined as follows in the Bateman classification:
- Small tear (<1 cm)
- Medium-size tear (1–3 cm)
- Large tear (3–5 cm)
- Massive tear (>5 cm)

Cuff tears can also be classified by their shape: Longitudinal, transverse, stellate, or massive.

Management of Partial Tear

Partial rotator cuff tears which are usually associated with adhesive capsulitis, are mostly treated symptomatically with corticosteroid injections to reduce the irritation of the subacromial bursa.

The following factors suggest a favorable response to nonoperative treatment:
- Gradual onset of complaints
- Degenerative lesion
- Sedentary patient
- Advanced age
- Lack of motivation
- Concomitant limitation of motion (e.g., frozen shoulder)

Conservative treatment includes analgesic therapy combined with non-steroidal anti-inflammatory medication. A brief period of immobilization can be beneficial in the acute stage. Subacromial corticosteroid injection will reduce acute pain symptoms but should not be done more than three times, as this would compromise the prognosis of a subsequent operative repair.

As a rule, intensive physical therapy program is initiated to strengthen the rotators and adductors, as these muscles will bring the humeral head downward (depressors) and thus restore dynamic equilibrium between the deltoid muscle and rotator cuff. Distal movement of the humeral head will also expand the narrowed subacromial space. If conservative treatment does not yield the desired result, arthoroscopic subacromial decompression (ASD) should be performed. Subacromial bursectomy and acromioplasty causing mechanical problems are usually helpful in reducing the symptoms.

If the partial tear involves >50% of the tendon thickness and there is a history of an acute event, rotator cuff repair may be considered.

Unfavorable factors are advanced age, large cuff defect, passive limitation of shoulder motion due to arthritis, small acromiohumeral distance, cuff tears in zone A or in all three zones, and obesity.

■ OPERATIVE TECHNIQUE (FIGS. 10 TO 17)

Position

Rotator cuff repair can be done in both beach chair and lateral position. Each one has its advantage and disadvantage. We prefer lateral position. Patient's head is fixed to the table with cushioning on eyes and ears to avoid injury while handling the instruments. Pillow is placed below head to avoid lateral pull to the brachial plexus.

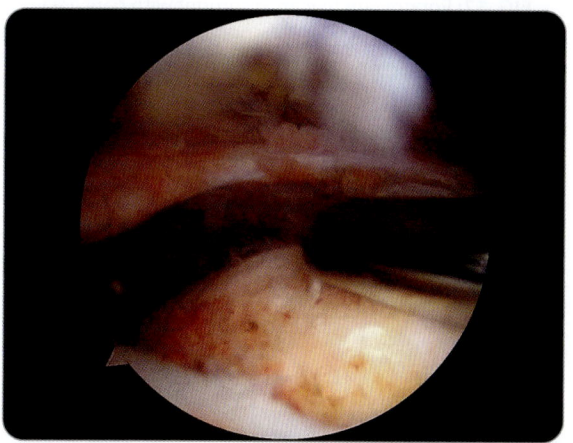

FIG. 10: Rotator cuff tear and footprint.

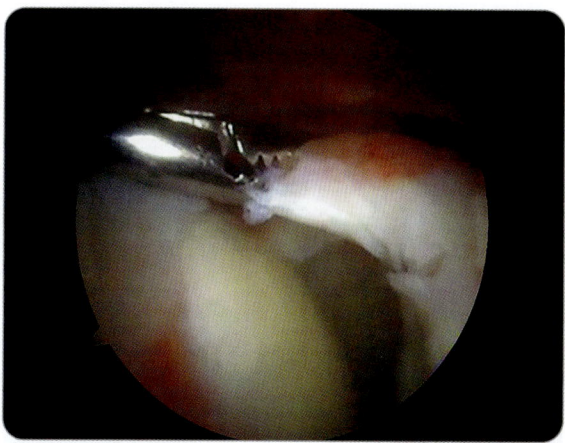

FIG. 11: Assessing retractability of the cuff.

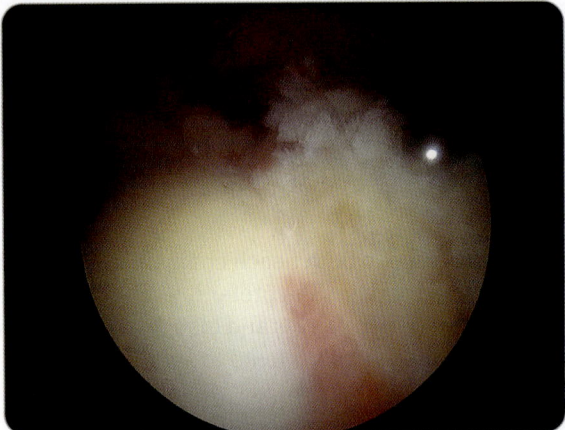

FIG. 12: Rotator cuff tear and footprint with bare area.

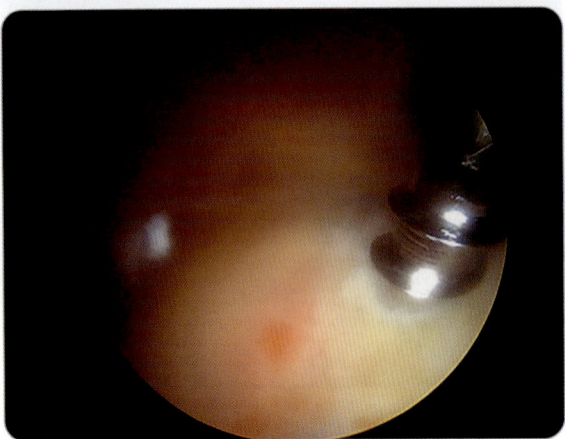

FIG. 13: Placing entry owl for PEEK anchor.

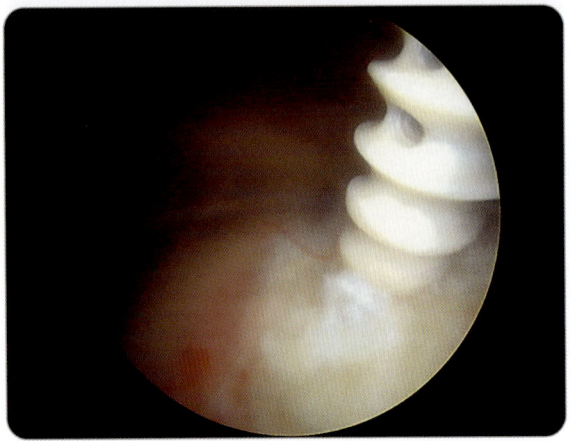

FIG. 14: Placing the suture anchor.

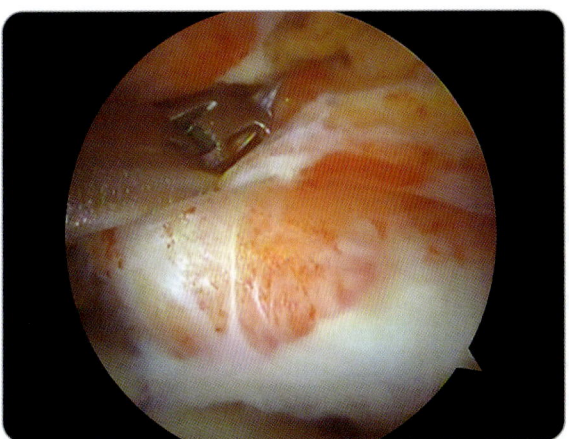

FIG. 15: Taking bites in the rotator cuff.

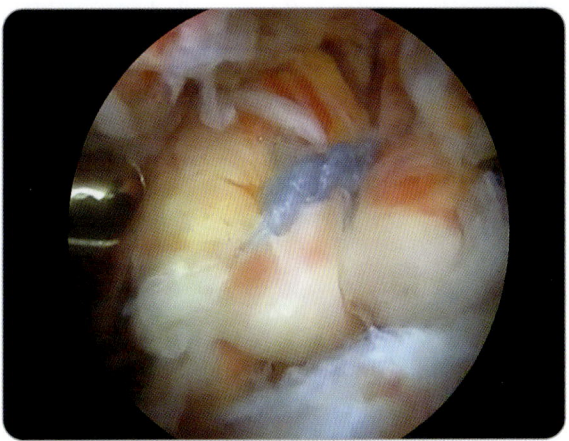

FIG. 16: Rotator cuff after tying the suture knots.

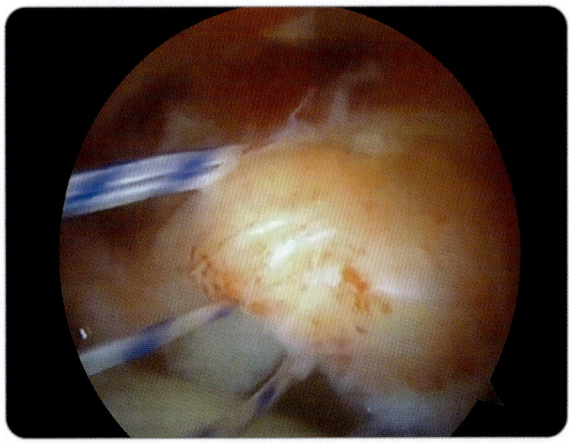

FIG. 17: Taken bite in the cuff.

Portals

Standard posterior portal, postaro-lateral portal as viewing portal. Anterosuperior and lateral portal as working portals.

Diagnostic arthroscopy is done using posterior portal. Lateral portal is taken 3 cm lateral to the edge of acromion. An 8-mm plastic cannula is passed after dilating the portal. Anterosuperior portal with 6 mm cannula is used as an accessory working portal for suture management. Using posterolateral viewing portal as bird's eye view, subacromial bursectomy is done using shaver in the posterior and subdeltoid region.

Hemostasis is achieved with radio frequency ablator. Undersurface of anterolateral acromion is decompressed with 4 mm burr to avoid impingement of the repaired cuff. Once adequate space is created in the subacromial region, assessment of rotator cuff and bicep tendon pathology is done with the help of probe and grasper. The degenerated edges of the cuff are debrided, and biceps tenotomy is performed if found shredded. If biceps is in good condition, it can be used as adjuvant in massive rotator cuff tears called reverse biceps tenodesis or biceps SCR.

Types of Tear

- Crescent shaped
- "U" shaped
- "L" shaped
- Reverse "L" shaped

Footprint Preparation

Footprint of cuff insertion on the greater tuberosity is debrided with the help of shaver and burr to achieve pinpoint bleeding. Care is taken not to violate the cortex. Depending upon the size of the tear, the number of anchors and their positioning is planned. For double row repair, medial row anchors are placed just lateral to the cartilage of humeral head. If even after release, cuff is coming up to the humeral head, medialization of the footprint can be done by removing 4 mm of cartilage of humeral head. Anchor hold is much better in the subchondral region and near the bicipital tuberosity.

Anchor Placement

With the help of spinal needle along the lateral edge of the acromion, direction of anchor insertion is assessed. Once satisfied, small stab incision is made close to the lateral edge of acromion. A variety of anchors are available such as 2.8 mm all-suture anchor and 5.5 mm anchors [bioabsorbable, polyether-ether-ketone (PEEK), and titanium] are available. Depending upon the bone quality at the footprint, anchors are chosen. For osteoporotic bone, 6 mm metal anchors are preferred. All-suture anchors which expand under the cortex have the advantage of smaller bone tunnels and lesser bone loss. After inserting the double-loaded anchor at desired marking of the inserter, handle is removed. One suture is pulled out of the lateral portal, and rest are parked in the anterosuperior portal. For anterior and lateral part of the repair, antegrade device like scorpion is used through the lateral portal to take bites through the rotator cuff at the depth of 15 mm. For posterior part of the tear like infraspinatus, retrograde suture passing devices like bird beak or suture lasso are used for better width of the tendon. Care is taken to avoid bites through the muscular part of the cuff to avoid cut-through. The sutures coming out of the rotator cuff are parked in the AS portal. Procedure is repeated for remaining sutures sequentially to avoid confusion while tying the knots. Same procedure is repeated with the second anchor 8 mm apart.

Suture configuration: For single-row repair, combination of Mason–Allen and simple suture is preferred. For double-row repair, mattress configuration is preferred. In double-row repair, multiple options have evolved like transosseous repair, transosseous equivalent, and linked (medial knot-tying) and nonlinked (no medial knots) double-row repair.

Knot-tying: Authors prefer SMC sliding knot, as it is self-locking and less bulky than others. Sequence of knot-tying is from posterior to anterior. For "U"-shaped tears, margin conversion sutures are used to close the anterior and posterior flaps followed by suturing the lateral margin of the cuff. For double-row repair, the lateral-row sutures are fixed with a knotless anchor 10 mm lateral to the medial-row anchors.

Suture material: Traditionally, high strength polyethylene sutures (No. 2) such as fiber-wire and orthocord are used. Recently, 1.5 mm suture tapes are preferred during double-row repair to avoid cheese cutting effect of the tendon (type 2 failure or retear).

POSTOPERATIVE CARE

If the cuff has been repaired without tension, the arm is immobilized in a Gilchrist bandage for 6 weeks. If the cuff was repaired under tension, a shoulder abduction splint may have to be worn for 4–6 weeks.

SUGGESTED READINGS

1. Strobel MJ (Ed). Manual of Arthroscopic Surgery. Berlin: Springer; 2002. pp. 886-9.
2. Strobel MJ (Ed). Manual of Arthroscopic Surgery. Berlin: Springer; 2002. pp. 917-26.
3. Burkhart SS, Lo IKY, Brady PC. Visualization. In: Burkhart SS, Lo IKY, Brady PC (Eds). Burkhart's View of the Shoulder: A Cowboy's Guide to Advanced Shoulder Arthroscopy. Philadelphia: Lippincott Williams and Wilkins; 2006. pp. 249-87.

Anterior Instability

Vaibhav J Koli, Aditya R Gunjotikar, Rohit Mahesh Sane, Shivam Mehra

■ CAUSES

Direct or indirect violence can cause the humeral head to dislocate from the glenoid. A critical factor is whether the dislocation was caused by adequate trauma or a particular movement. Differentiating between a traumatic and non-traumatic etiology has an important bearing on further management.

■ CLASSIFICATION

Frequency: An initial dislocation is distinguished from recurrent dislocation.

Etiology: The dislocation is classified as having a traumatic or atraumatic etiology. Factors that suggest a traumatic etiology are as follows: history of an adequate traumatic event, lengthy delay between dislocation and reduction, shoulder can only be reduced under general anesthesia, presence of a bony Bankart lesion, and presence of a large Hill–Sachs lesion.

The following factors are more consistent with an atraumatic etiology: increased ligamentous laxity, no history of adequate trauma, proneness to dislocation, spontaneous reduction, shoulder can be reduced without general anesthesia, and absence of a Hill–Sachs lesion.

Direction of the dislocation: The humeral head may dislocate anteriorly, posteriorly, or inferiorly.

■ SYMPTOMS

In most traumatic initial shoulder dislocations, spontaneous reduction is not possible. The patient describes very severe pain involving the entire shoulder and sometimes the entire arm. Patients with an existing shoulder instability and a history of inadequate trauma or an inciting movement describe less pain. In these cases, a helper or even the patient himself can reduce the dislocation by gently pulling on the arm.

CHAPTER 11: Anterior Instability

■ CLINICAL DIAGNOSIS (FIGS. 1 TO 3)

Given the major therapeutic implications of the etiology, a detailed evaluation is necessary. It must be determined whether the dislocation is traumatic or atraumatic.

Acute anterior dislocation: The arm is held in a position of slight abduction, anteversion, and external rotation. The patient complains of very severe pain. The contour of the shoulder may or may not differ from the unaffected side. In some cases, the examiner can palpate the empty glenoid and the dislocated humeral head, which is next to or below the coracoid process. Blood flow (radial artery) and sensation (axillary nerve) should always be tested. If tests indicate neurovascular compromise, the shoulder should be reduced immediately after the radiographic examination.

Recurrent dislocation: The patient gives a prior history of an initial dislocation. It is important to establish whether the prior dislocation could be easily reduced (e.g., by a helper pulling on the arm) or whether it required reduction under general anesthesia. The latter indicates a traumatic etiology of the initial dislocation.

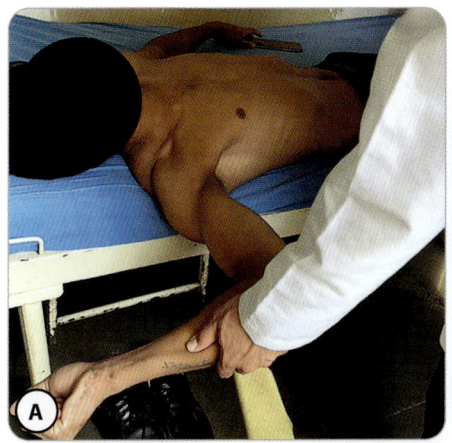
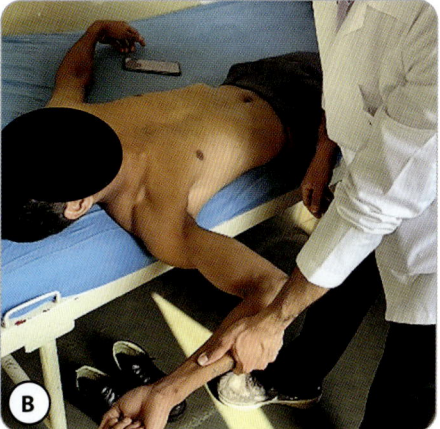
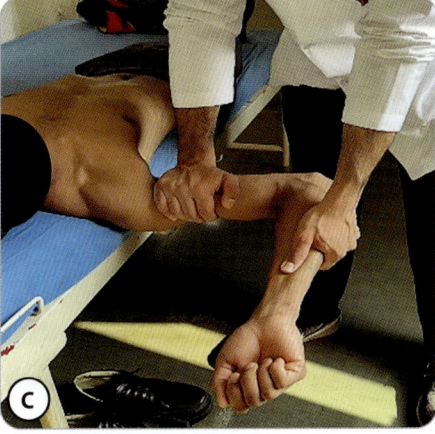

FIGS. 1A TO C: (A) Apprehension test; (B) Relocation test; (C) Release test.

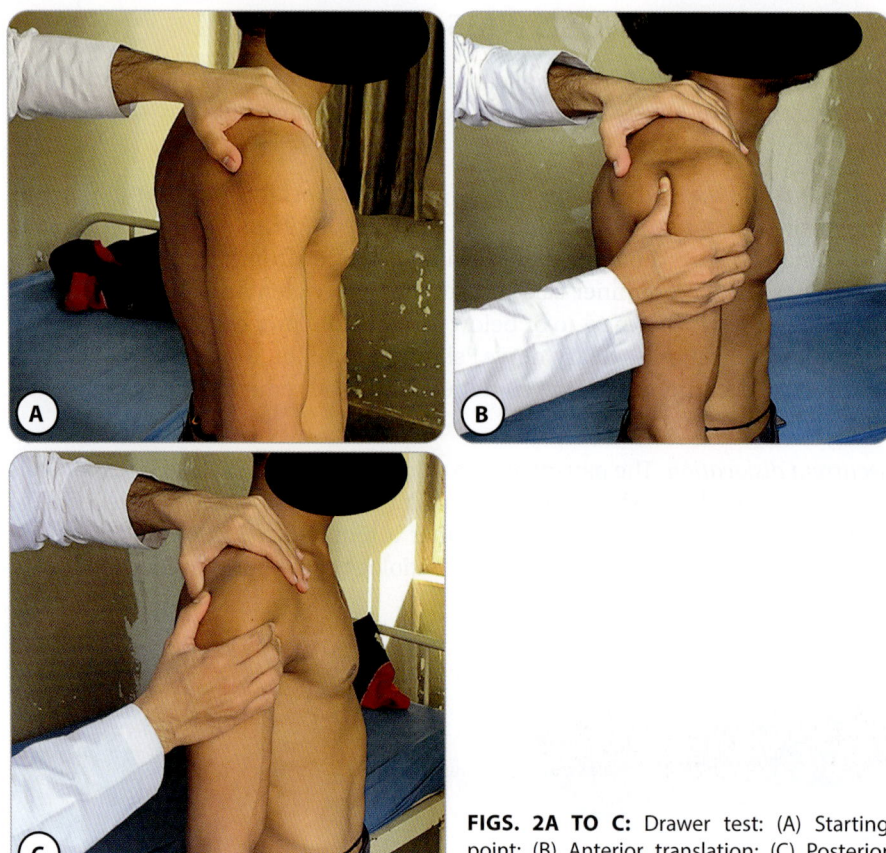

FIGS. 2A TO C: Drawer test: (A) Starting point; (B) Anterior translation; (C) Posterior translation.

FIGS. 3A AND B: Sulcus sign: (A) Starting position; (B) Ending position.

Following recurrent dislocations, the joint is usually found to be in a reduced rather than dislocated position. Often the dislocation is easily reduced with traction applied by a helper or the patient himself. Usually, the range of shoulder motion is undiminished. The anterior apprehension test consists of abduction and external rotation of the shoulder. A positive test elicits muscular guarding to keep the shoulder from dislocating or subluxating anteriorly **(Figs. 1A to C)**.

General ligamentous laxity should be tested as well. A positive sulcus sign on both sides (inferior displacement of the humerus by downward traction on the relaxed forearm) indicates general ligamentous laxity. Unilateral multidirectional instability results in a unilateral positive sulcus sign **(Figs. 3A and B)**.

Radiographs

Dislocated position: Radiographs in two planes (AP view and scapular Y view) document the dislocated position and exclude fractures of the humeral head and glenoid **(Fig. 4A)**.

Reduced position: Radiographs in the reduced position can demonstrate secondary changes in the glenoid, such as an osseous Bankart lesion and a Hill–Sachs lesion in the humeral head **(Fig. 4B)**.

Avulsion fractures of the greater tuberosity can also be excluded **(Fig. 4C)**.

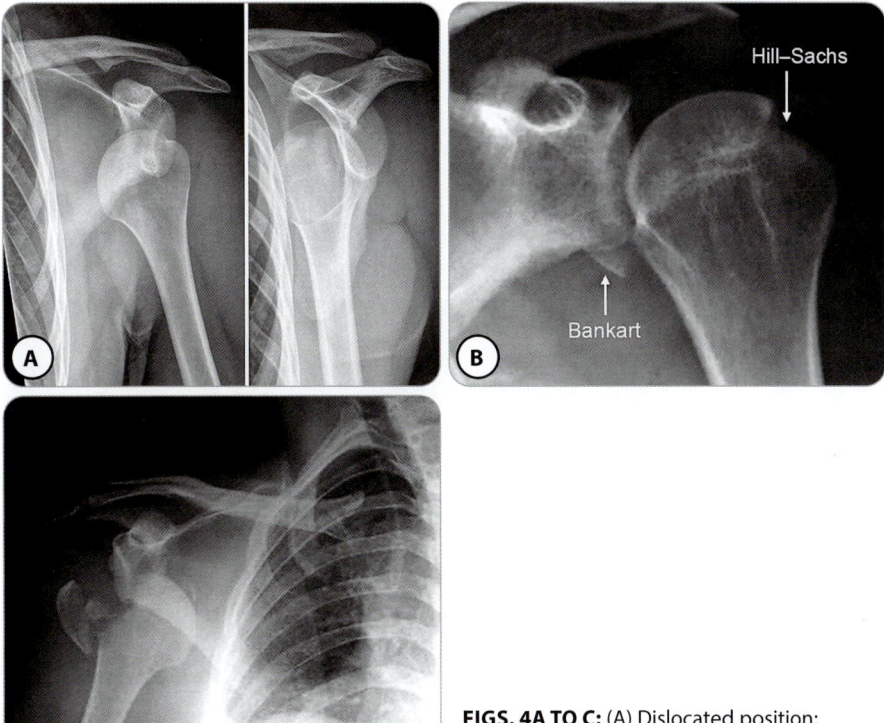

FIGS. 4A TO C: (A) Dislocated position; (B) Secondary changes in the glenoid; and (C) Avulsion fractures of the greater tuberosity.

Ultrasound

A Hill–Sachs defect can be clearly visualized with ultrasound. The shoulder is also scanned for rotator cuff lesions, since partial and full-thickness tears can accompany shoulder dislocation, especially in patients over 40 years of age. Rotator cuff repairs are of special importance in these cases.

Magnetic Resonance Imaging and Computed Tomography (Figs. 5A to D)

Magnetic resonance imaging (MRI) or double-contrast computed tomography (CT) scanning is recommended for preoperative planning, especially if an arthroscopic repair is proposed. These studies are helpful for evaluating the condition of the anterior capsule, glenoid rim, and labrum and excluding pre-existing torsional deformity of the humerus.

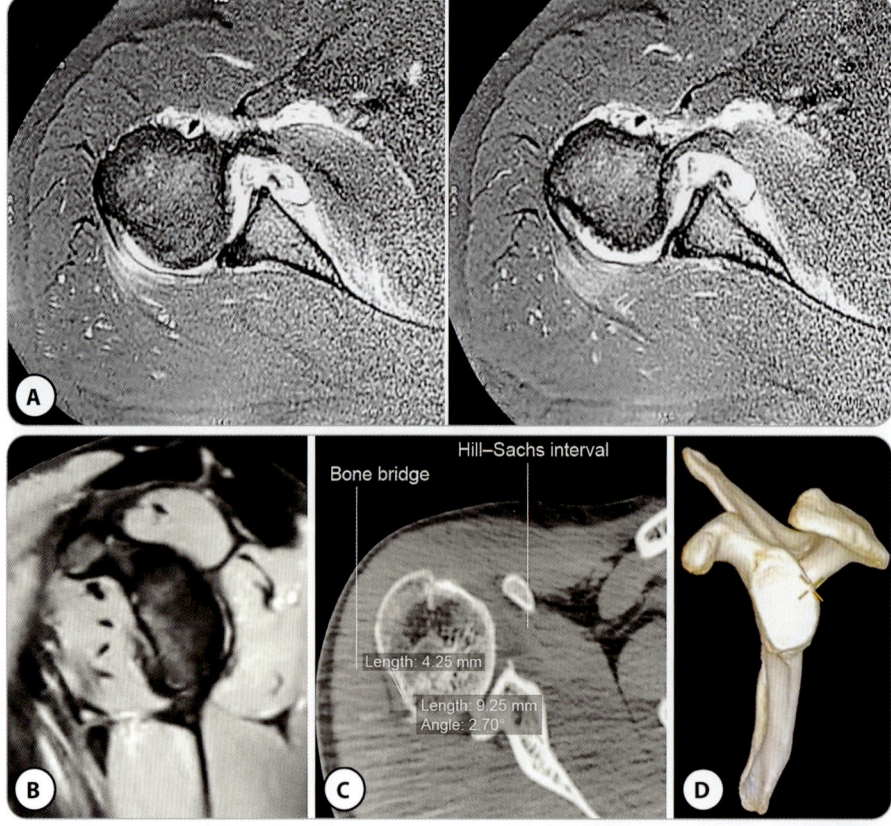

FIGS. 5A TO D: (A) MRI images of anterior labral tear; (B) CT image of loss of anterior glenoid bone; (C) Calculating HS index; and (D) 3D-CT image of loss of anterior glenoid bone.
(CT: computed tomography; MRI: magnetic resonance imaging)

Arthroscopic Findings

There are a number of characteristic intra-articular changes that differ from normal findings.

Bankart lesion **(Fig. 6)**: This lesion involves a detachment of the anterior–inferior labrum from the glenoid with involvement of the inferior glenohumeral ligament. The continuity between the cartilage and labrum is disrupted, but the periosteal attachment is intact. Areas of interstitial hemorrhage may be seen after acute injuries, while recurrent dislocations may present with degenerative fraying of the labrum and occasional labral tears.

Hill–Sachs lesion **(Fig. 7)**: This lesion consists of a chondral or osteochondral impaction in the posterolateral aspect of the humeral head. The Hill–Sachs defect

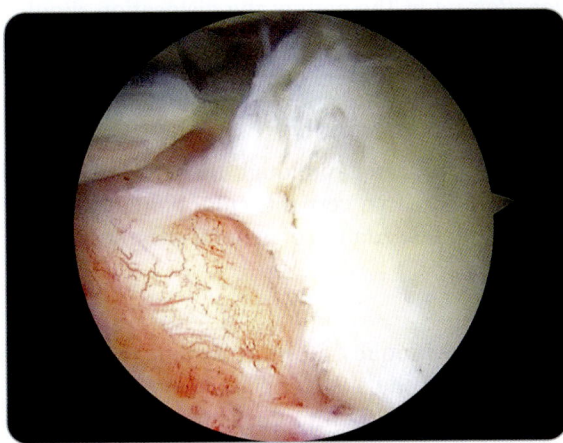

FIG. 6: Bankart lesion.

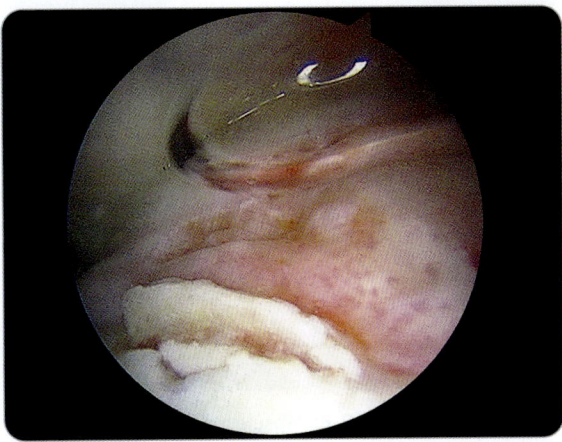

FIG. 7: Hill–Sachs lesion.

is typically V shaped. If the dislocation is reproduced during arthroscopy, the configuration of the defect matches the anterior labrum–glenoid complex.

Glenoid lesions: These injuries affect the anterior-inferior region of the glenoid. They range from chondral flake fractures to anteroinferior glenoid fractures. Extensive cartilage lesions with degenerative fraying of the labrum signify numerous prior dislocations joint space (chronic anterior instability).

Capsular lesions **(Fig. 8)**: Tearing of the inferior glenohumeral ligament may occur, even if the labrum remains firmly attached to the glenoid. Combined injuries involving the anterior inferior labrum can also occur.

Associated lesions: Intra-articular loose bodies may consist of chondral fragments sheared from the glenoid or fragments from a Hill–Sachs lesion. Partial or full-thickness rotator cuff tears should also be excluded.

Finding the dislocation path: The path of the dislocation should be reproduced under arthroscopic control to establish the direction of the dislocation.

■ THERAPEUTIC MANAGEMENT

Immediate reduction is indicated, although this can be quite difficult with an initial traumatic dislocation. In a very muscular patient, it may be necessary to perform the reduction under sedation or general anesthesia.

Reduction

In the classic reduction techniques, an effort is made to manipulate the humeral head—which is engaged on the anterior glenoid rim by a Hill-Sachs lesion and fixed by muscular guarding—back into the glenoid fossa. The reduction should be accomplished carefully and "without force." In principle, the humeral head is freed from its dislocated position using traction and an axillary fulcrum, externally

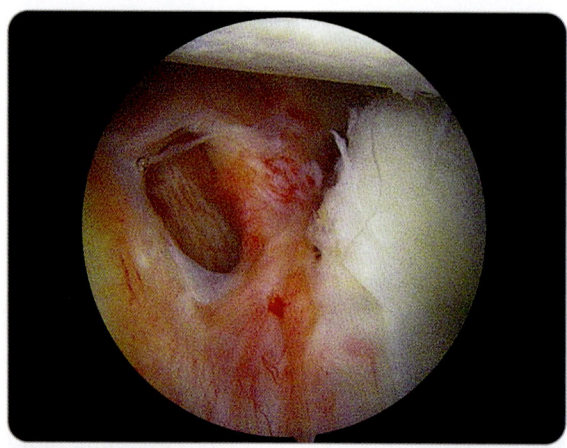

FIG. 8: Capsule rent.

rotated, and then reduced in internal rotation. The axillary fulcrum may consist of a heel (Hippocratic technique), fist (Milch technique), or chair back (Arlt technique). In the Stimson technique, the patient lies in a prone position and hangs the affected arm over the edge of the examination table. A weight or manual traction is then placed on the arm to induce gradual muscular relaxation. This is supported by repeatedly telling the patient to relax the muscles throughout the procedure. It may take up to 20–30 minutes for spontaneous reduction to occur.

After the dislocation has been reduced, whether under anesthesia or using one of the techniques described, blood flow and sensation are again tested and biplane radiographs are obtained. If a glenoid or humeral head fracture is suspected, an extra radiographic view or preferably CT scans should be obtained to document the extent of the fracture.

CONSERVATIVE TREATMENT

Following an initial dislocation, the shoulder is first immobilized. It has been found that immobilizing the shoulder for longer than 3 weeks does not decrease the rate of re-dislocation. Physical therapy is then initiated to increase the range of motion. Rotator- and adductor-strengthening exercises are also performed. Generally, this treatment is less successful for posttraumatic instabilities than atraumatic instabilities.

OPERATIVE TECHNIQUE

Recurrent Anterior Instability

Studies by Bankart proved that a labrum that has been detached by a dislocation will not heal spontaneously in a normal position. The incidence of recurrence after an initial dislocation will vary, depending on the etiology (traumatic or atraumatic). Given the complex anatomy of the shoulder joint and the various types of lesions and associated injuries that can occur, more than 150 different operative techniques have been devised for the treatment of recurrent anterior shoulder dislocation. Two basic types of operative techniques are available (Wiedemann, 1996):
1. *Anatomic techniques*: The goal of these techniques is to produce an anatomic reconstruction of the damaged structures.
2. *Palliative techniques*: These techniques involve creating or surgically introducing a barrier to prevent recurrent dislocation. Examples are the Latarjet procedure, the Lange bone graft procedure, and the Eden–Hybinette procedure.

Indications

An essential criterion in selecting patients for operative treatment is the high incidence of re-dislocations in the presence of coexisting labral injuries. Re-dislocation rates of 60–90% have been reported in the literature.

In selecting a suitable anatomic reconstruction, it must be decided whether to use arthroscopic or open technique. This has become a frequent topic of discussion at every scientific conference that deals with shoulder instability.

For the present, therefore, we must weigh the advantages and disadvantages of arthroscopic techniques and draw our own conclusions:

Advantages:
- Low invasiveness
- No risk to proprioception

Disadvantages:
- Complex operative technique
- Increased complication rate when metallic implants are used
- Need for a posterior incision when transglenoid fixation is used
- Higher incidence of recurrence

Contraindications to Arthroscopic Repair

Each of the following factors would contraindicate an arthroscopic procedure:
- Bony Bankart lesion
- Hill–Sachs defect
- Absence or destruction of the labrum–capsule–ligament complex (e.g., Quatro labral lesion)
- *Associated lesions*: While technically these lesions would not preclude an arthroscopic repair, their presence would compromise a successful outcome:
  - Complete rupture of the subscapularis tendon
  - Interval lesion with subluxation or dislocation of the long biceps tendon
  - Tear of the subscapularis tendon
  - Multidirectional instability
  - Isolated posterior instability

Three-point Labral Repair: The Habermeyer Technique

This transglenoid technique is a modification of the Morgan repair.

Inspection and probing: The glenohumeral joint is visualized. The anterior-inferior labrum–capsule–ligament complex is carefully palpated with the probe through an anterior-inferior portal. Associated lesions (loose bodies, biceps tendon lesions, and rotator cuff tears) that might contraindicate an arthroscopic procedure are excluded. If the labrum–capsule–ligament complex is stable and there is no instability in another direction, it is feasible to proceed with arthroscopic repair. The portals are switched (arthroscope to an anterior portal), and the posterior joint region is inspected.

Removal of adhesions: Adhesions that have formed between the avulsed labrum and the scapular neck are removed with a cautery probe (hook electrode), basket forceps, or synovial resector. Dissection with the cautery probe should not be carried far distally along the scapular neck, as this might injure the axillary nerve.

If vision is inadequate, therefore, the adhesions should be removed with a basket forceps or rasp using a combination of blunt and sharp dissection.

Mobilizing the inferior glenohumeral ligament: This most important ligamentous component of the anterior capsular complex should be mobilized so that it can be raised to the level of the glenoid surface. According to Habermeyer (1996), the mobility of the labrum–ligament complex is critical to the success of this repair.

Freshening the anterior-inferior scapular neck: The scapular neck is decorticated with a curved sharp rasp or small round bur until a cancellous bed is obtained.

Placing the fixation sutures and anchor knots: A cannulated grasper is introduced and is used to grasp, elevate, tighten, and shorten the mobilized glenohumeral ligament. At the same time, the labrum is anatomically reduced to the glenoid rim. First the inferior glenohumeral ligament is grasped at its junction with the labrum and brought up to the 4 o'clock position (right shoulder) on the glenoid rim. Care is taken to achieve adequate tensioning the ligament.

Next, a pointed wire (1.7 mm in diameter) with an eyelet is introduced through the cannulated grasper and drilled into the glenoid rim at the junction of the cartilage and bone. The drilling angle is 30° inferior and 15° posteromedial relative to the scapular plane. The wire should enter the infraspinous fossa and exit the skin posteriorly about 10 cm below the scapular spine. A pair of sutures [polydioxanone suture (PDS)] is threaded through the eyelet in the wire, and the wire is pulled out posteriorly, bringing the sutures with it. The sutures are tied together to form an anchor knot approximately 4 mm in diameter. The suture tails protruding from the cannulated grasper are then pulled, drawing the anchor knot back through the skin and against the posterior scapula. The knot on the posterior scapular neck provides a stable posterior fixation point.

The same technique is used to drill a second transglenoid hole, parallel to the first, at the 3 o'clock position on the glenoid (lateral decubitus position). As before, a cannulated grasper is used and the Kirschner wire is brought out posteriorly with the second pair of sutures. The subcutaneous tissue is spread open, and the anchor knot is pulled back against the posterior scapular neck.

The advantage of the three-point suturing technique of Habermeyer is that it places stable anchor knots on the posterior scapular neck that will not loosen postoperatively as swelling subsides.

Anterior fixation: At this point, four sutures pass through the working cannula in the anterior portal. The sutures from the first transglenoid drill hole are clamped to distinguish them from the second suture pair. Under no circumstances should the two sutures from the first hole be tied together on the labrum. Instead, one of the superior sutures is matched to an inferior suture, and those sutures are tied together. A knot pusher is used to advance the knot through the cannula to the reduced labrum–capsule–ligament complex. The knot-tying technique should be clean and precise. Because the suture material is PDS, a minimum of five knots should be tied, and preferably six. The suture ends are trimmed with a small punch. The same technique is used to tie the two remaining sutures together and advance the knot.

Probing: The reattached labrum–ligament complex is palpated with the probe to assess the adequacy of the repair. Optimally, the labrum should be positioned over the glenoid rim so that it once again reinforces the anterior–inferior glenoid rim and enlarges the articular surface.

Caspari Technique of Arthroscopic Labral Repair

- Inspection and probing
- *Removal of adhesions*: As in the Habermeyer technique, adhesions between the avulsed labrum and scapular neck are removed.
- Mobilizing the inferior glenohumeral ligament
- Freshening the anterior–inferior scapular neck
- *Placing the fixation sutures*: The detached labrum–ligament complex is grasped as far inferiorly as possible with a special suture forceps called a Caspari suture punch. PDS suture material is advanced through the suture punch with a feeder mechanism until it appears within the joint. This technique is very similar to the all-inside technique for meniscal repairs.
- A total of 5–8 sutures are placed in the avulsed structures and brought out through an anterior instrument portal. Then a transglenoid hole is drilled with a 3.5-mm pin, angling the drill exactly as in the three-point technique. Drilling is started at the 12 o'clock position, however. The sutures are threaded through the eyelet at the end of the pin and passed from anterior to posterior through the transglenoid drill hole. On the posterior side, the sutures are tensioned and tied over the infraspinous fascia.
- Probing the repair
- The advantage of the Caspari technique is that the steps in the procedure are clearly divided into (1) piercing the labrum, (2) transglenoid drilling, and (3) passing the sutures through the drill hole and tying them. The disadvantage is the postoperative loosening that will occur as extravasated fluid clears during the initial hours after surgery. We, therefore, recommend placing the knots as deeply and as close to the posterior scapular neck as possible.

Suture Anchor System

- *Instrumentation*: Besides specially designed suture anchors, the instrument set includes a special cannulated grasper used both for drilling the guidewire and for inserting the complete suture anchor. Because this technique is purely anterior and does not require transglenoid drilling, it does not risk injury to structures posterior to the scapular neck (the suprascapular nerve).
- Inspection and probing
- Removal of adhesions
- *Mobilizing the inferior glenohumeral ligament* **(Fig. 9)**: As in the transglenoid techniques, mobilization of the inferior glenohumeral ligament is of key importance.
- *Freshening the anterior inferior scapular neck* **(Fig. 10A)**: The anterior scapular neck is freshened with a sharp rasp or small round bur **(Fig. 10B)**.

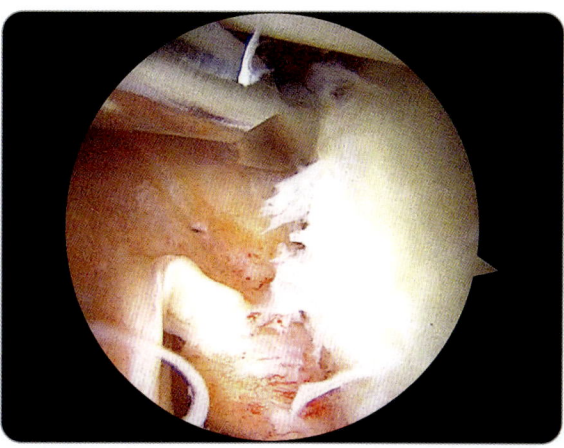

FIG. 9: Mobilizing the inferior glenohumeral ligament.

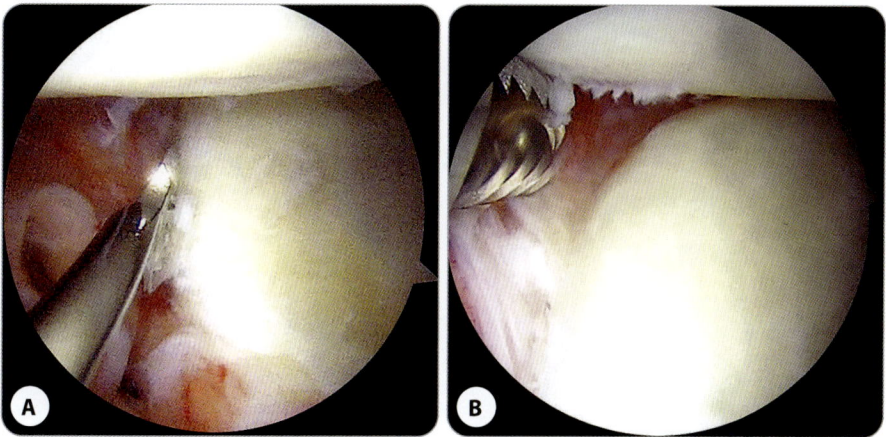

FIGS. 10A AND B: Freshening the anterior–inferior scapular neck.

- *Fixation of the labrum–ligament complex with the suture anchor*: The grasper is introduced through a working cannula in the anterior-superior portal and grasps the detached capsule ligament complex. The complex should be grasped securely and moved toward the biceps tendon. The grasper remains in place, and the suture anchor is twisted in through the grasper using a special applicator. It is mostly a No. 2 PDS suture **(Figs. 11 to 14A)**.
- The grasper is withdrawn, leaving the threaded anchor in place. A single suture loop passes from the anterior scapular neck through the avulsed labrum ligament complex. From there, it passes out of the joint through the working cannula. After the first suture anchor has been placed at the 5–5:30 o'clock position, a second suture anchor is placed at the 4 and 2 o'clock position using an identical technique **(Figs. 14B and C to 18)**.

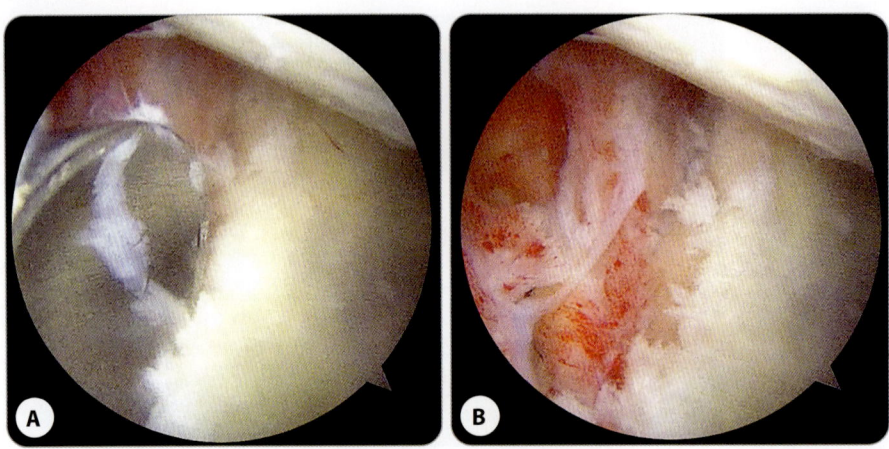

FIGS. 11A AND B: Preparing a healthy bleeding bed on the face of glenoid by removing cartilage rim with the help of curette.

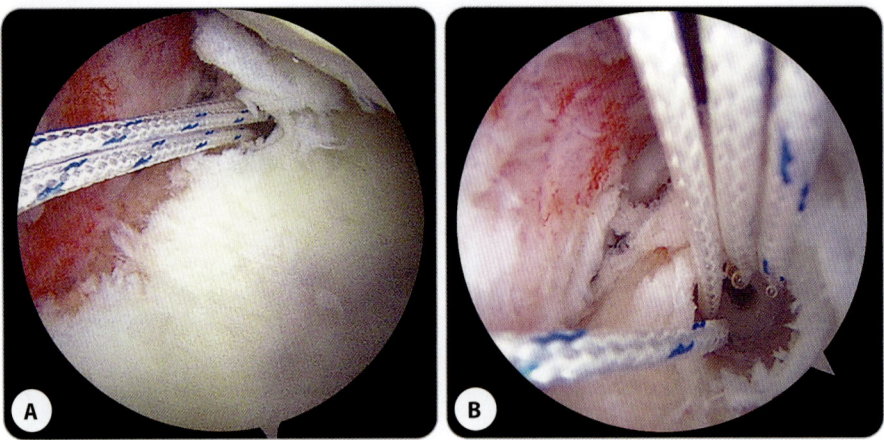

FIGS. 12A AND B: Insertion of suture anchor on the face of glenoid.

- Next the sutures are tied. The suture tails from the same anchor should not be tied together. This is avoided by tagging the tails from the first anchor with a hemostat or small knot. The knots are advanced to the anterior capsule with a knot pusher.

Mitek Anchor System

- *Instrumentation*: The instrument set includes a special drill bit matched to the length and diameter of the suture anchor. A special drill sleeve is required along with an inserter for the suture anchor. Also required are a suture passing instrument and suture passing tips with assorted angulations. As an alternative, the all-inside meniscal repair set can be used.

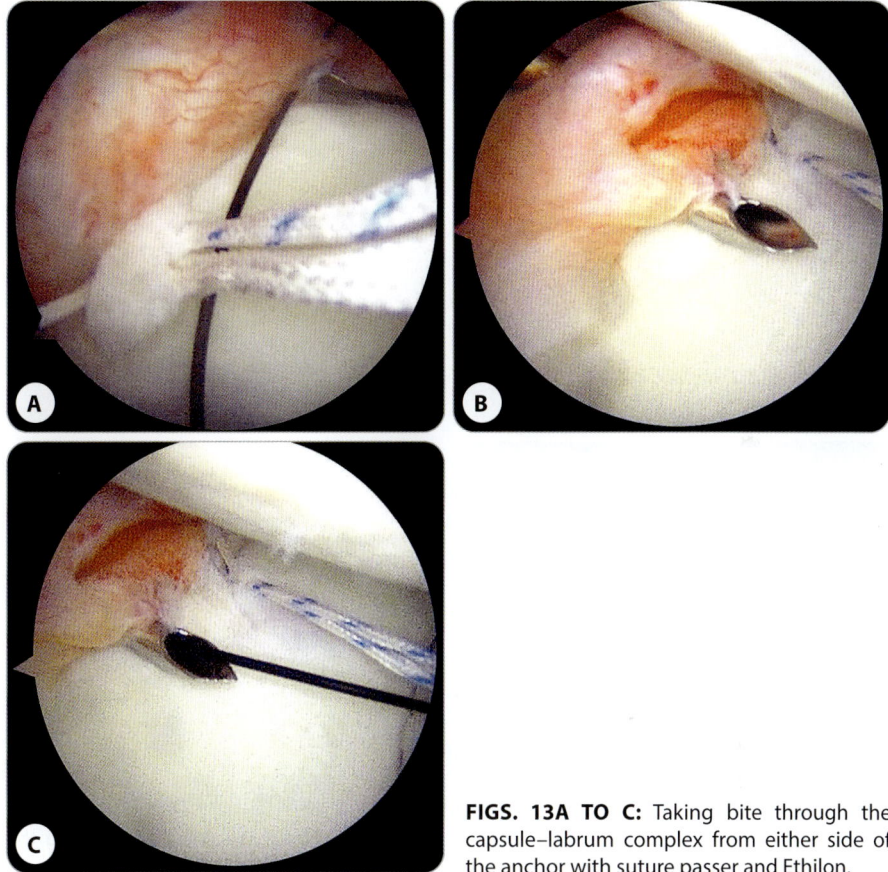

FIGS. 13A TO C: Taking bite through the capsule–labrum complex from either side of the anchor with suture passer and Ethilon.

- Inspection and probing
- Removal of adhesions
- Mobilizing the inferior glenohumeral ligament
- Freshening the anterior–inferior scapular neck
- *Drilling pilot holes for the suture anchors*: A special "shark-mouth" drill sleeve is introduced through the anterior–inferior portal and positioned at the bone cartilage junction of the glenoid. Usually, three pilot holes are drilled. The first hole is placed as low on the anterior glenoid as possible, and the second hole is placed as high as possible. The third hole is placed between the first two. The holes should be drilled at a 15–20° posterior angle relative to the glenoid surface.
- *Suturing the capsulolabral complex*: The suture hook is introduced through the working cannula and passed through the capsulolabral complex inferior to the highest of the pilot holes (see above). The suture is advanced through the hook and grasped with a small grasping forceps.

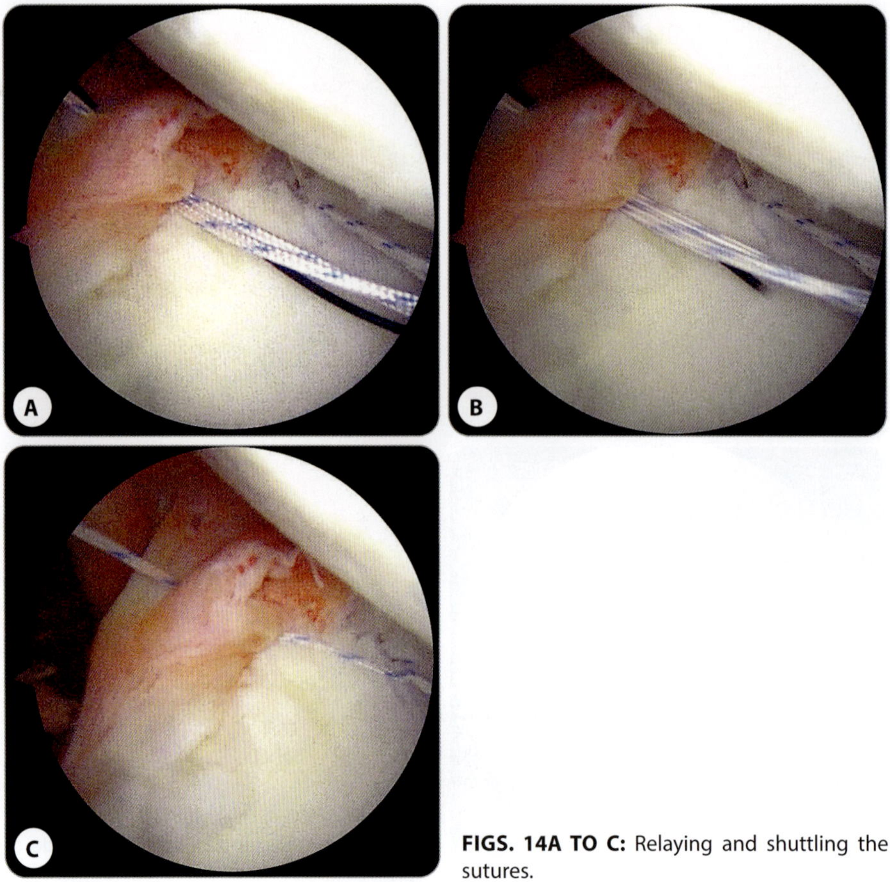

FIGS. 14A TO C: Relaying and shuttling the sutures.

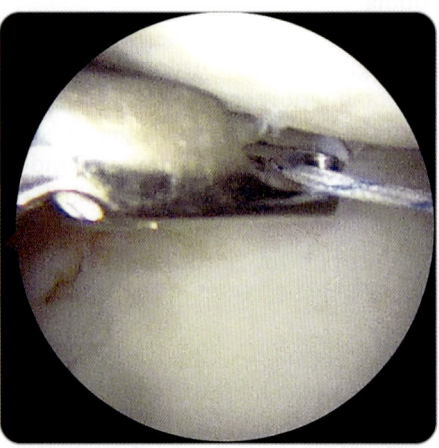

FIG. 15: Retrieving the other suture limb with suture retriever.

CHAPTER 11: Anterior Instability

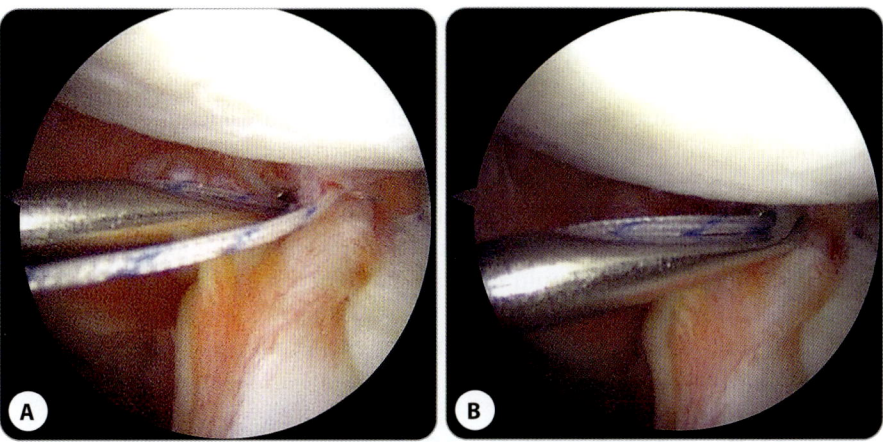

FIGS. 16A AND B: Knot tying.

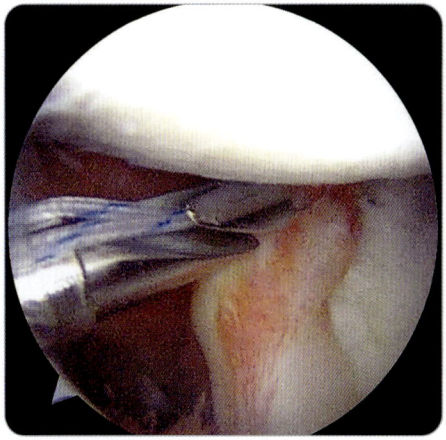

FIG. 17: Cutting the excess suture limbs with cutter.

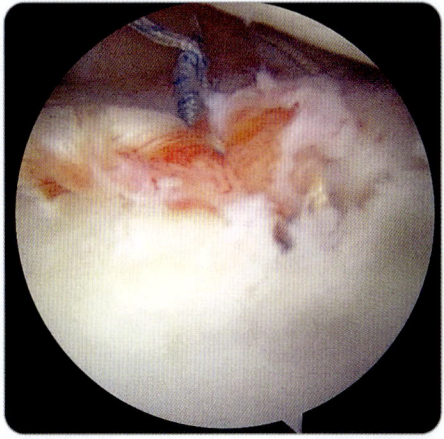

FIG. 18: Final picture of fixation of the capsule–labrum–ligament complex with the suture anchor.

- *Inserting the suture anchor*: Before the suture anchor is placed in the inserter, a fixation suture is passed through its eyelet to hold the anchor securely at the tip of the rod. The end of the suture that was placed through the capsulolabral complex is also threaded through the eyelet. The suture anchor is then passed through the working cannula into the joint space on the tip of the inserter, and the anchor is driven into the pilot hole.
- *Tying the sutures*: The two suture tails protruding from the working cannula are now tied together, and the knot is advanced into the joint with a knot pusher. The first knot should consist of a fisherman's slip knot. Then two square knots are tied over the slip knot and advanced to the repair site. Finally, the sutures are trimmed. The same technique is used to insert the remaining anchors.

Latarjet Reconstruction (Figs. 19 to 30)
- Make a deltopectoral incision.
- Identify the conjoined tendon and follow it proximally to the tip of the coracoid. At that point, identify the pectoralis minor attachment insertion into the medial aspect of the distal coracoid.
- Detach the pectoralis minor insertion from the medial coracoid with a pencil-tipped electrocautery probe.
- Detach the coracoacromial ligament from the lateral coracoid with electrocautery. With a periosteal elevator, clear the soft tissue circumferentially around the coracoid, which is now free of all soft tissue attachments (except for the conjoined tendon) from its tip to its base, where the coracoclavicular ligaments attach.
- Use an oscillating saw with a 70° angle blade to osteotomize the coracoid just anterior to the coracoclavicular ligaments. This will usually provide a coracoid bone graft 2.5–3 cm in length.

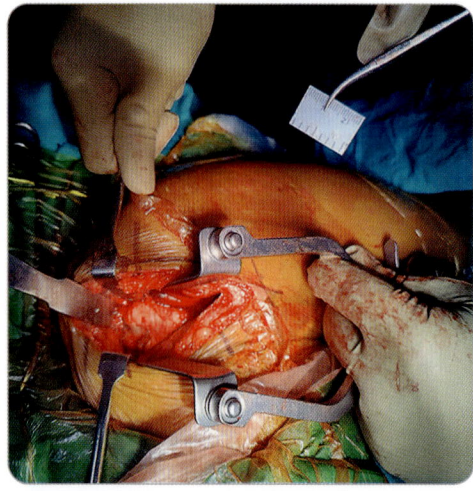

FIG. 19: Deltopectoral incision and identifying the conjoined tendon.

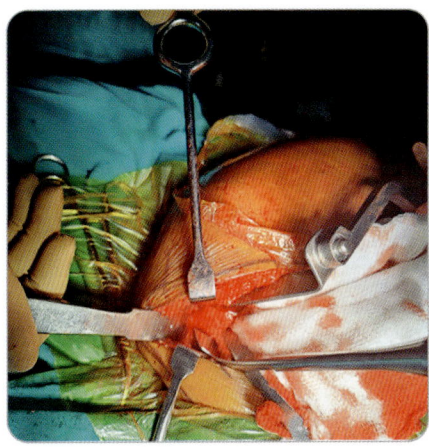

FIG. 20: Detaching the pectoralis minor insertion from the medial coracoid.

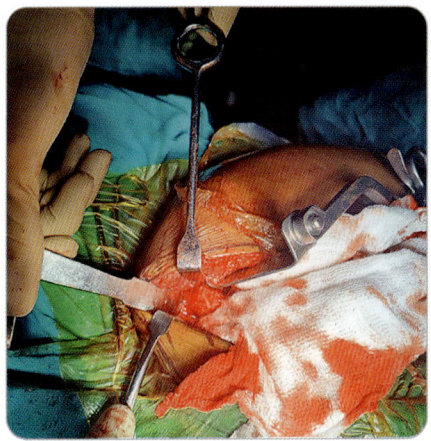

FIG. 21: Exposing the coracoid circumferentially.

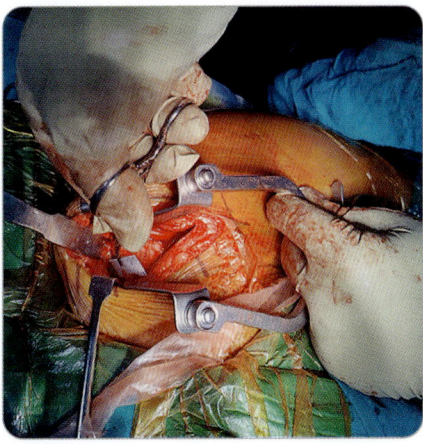

FIG. 22: Measuring the length of coracoid process.

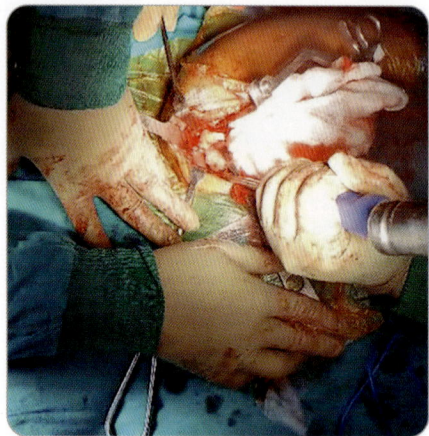

FIG. 23: Performing coracoid osteotomy with a curved osteotome.

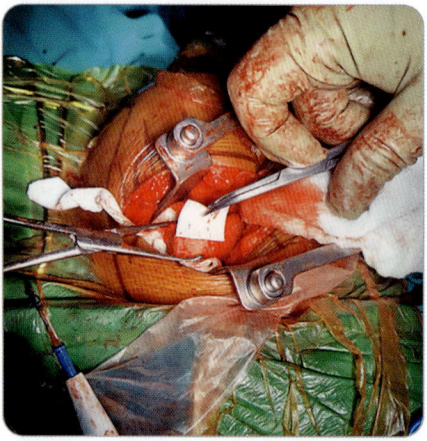

FIG. 24: Measuring the length of coracoid process obtained after osteotomy.

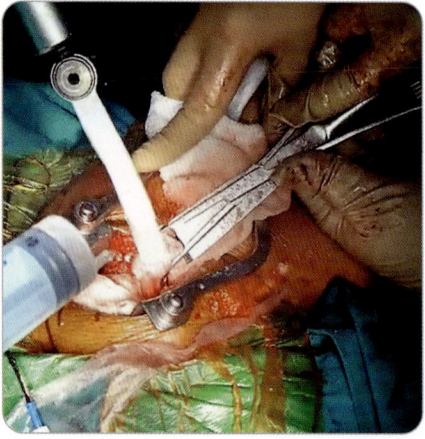

FIG. 25: Freshening the medial surface of the coracoid with an oscillating saw.

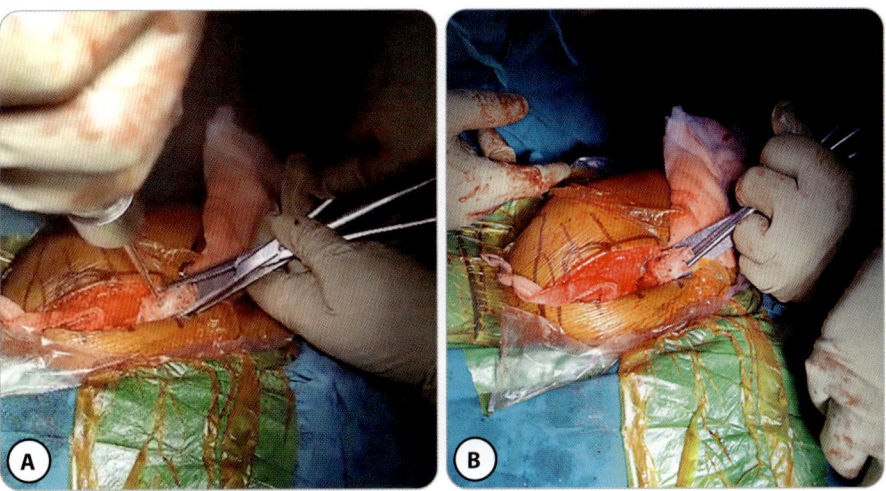

FIGS. 26A AND B: Drilling holes in coracoid process.

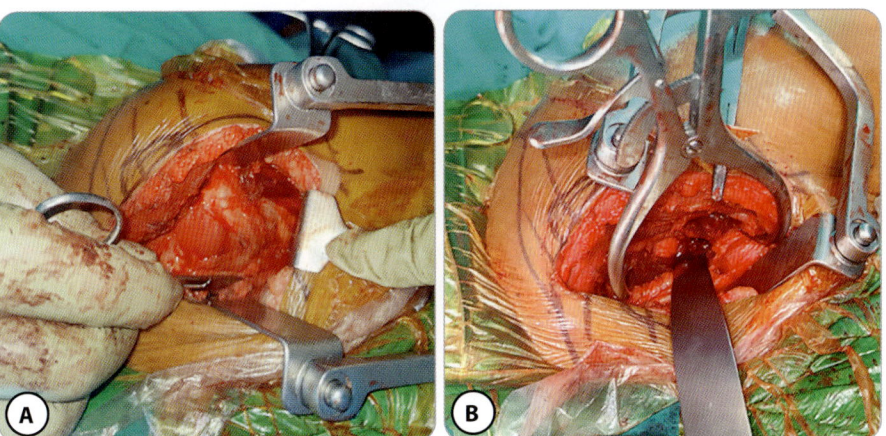

FIGS. 27A AND B: Splitting the subscapularis.

- Detach the upper half of the subscapularis distally and dissect it free from the underlying capsule. Then, develop the plane between the capsule and the lower half of the subscapularis tendon.
- Dissect an inverted L-shaped capsular flap, with the transverse limb of the inverted L at the level of the upper subscapularis tendon and the vertical limb of the L located 1 cm medial to the glenoid rim. Carry this flap down to the 6 o'clock position. A Fukuda ring retractor on the humeral head facilitates this dissection.
- The medial side of the coracoid graft is the side that will be placed against the glenoid. Prepare this medial side of the coracoid by freshening its surface with an oscillating saw.

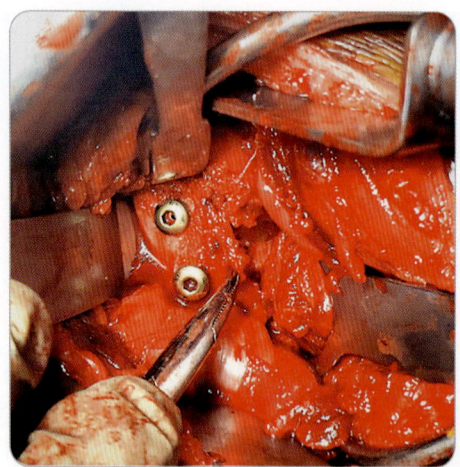

FIG. 28: Securing the graft with two 4.5-mm cannulated screws.

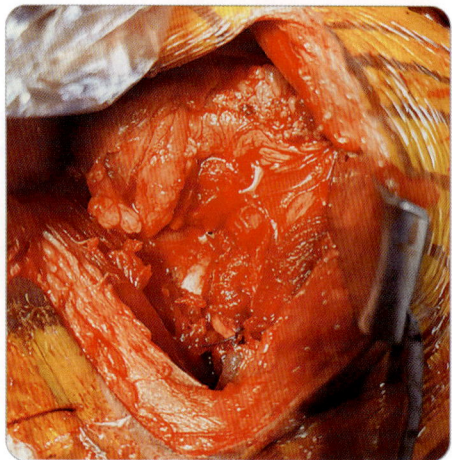

FIG. 29: Repairing the capsule.

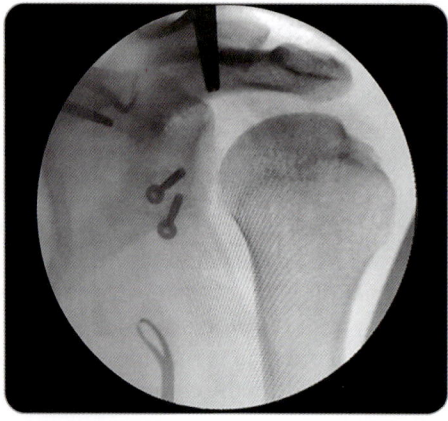

FIG. 30: Final C-arm picture.

- Then, with a burr, freshen the anterior glenoid neck to a bleeding base of bone.
- Place Bio-anchors in the anteroinferior rim of the native glenoid.
- Position the coracoid graft as an extension of the glenoid articular arc, provisionally holding it in place with two K-wires.
- Secure the graft with two 4.5-mm cannulated screws.
- Test the security of the construct.
- Repair the capsule with the sutures from the anchors in the glenoid. This repair ensures that the coracoid bone graft is extracapsular.
- Repair the upper subscapularis repaired to its anatomic position.

POSTOPERATIVE CARE

The shoulder is immobilized in a Gilchrist bandage for 6 weeks. Mobilization is begun in week 6, but external rotation and forcible abduction should be avoided until week 12. The patient should refrain from sports for 6 months.

SUGGESTED READINGS

1. Strobel MJ. Manual of arthroscopic surgery. Berlin: Springer; 2002. pp. 905-17.
2. Burkhart SS, Lo IKY, Brady PC. Visualization. In: Burkhart SS, Lo IKY, Brady PC (Eds). Burkhart's view of the shoulder. A cowboy's guide to advanced shoulder arthroscopy. Philadelphia: Lippincott Williams & Wilkins; 2006. pp. 223-6.

CHAPTER 12

Frozen Shoulder

Sachin Yashwant Kale, Anup Krishnan, Arvind J Vatkar, Aditya R Gunjotikar, Vishal Kumar

■ CAUSE

Frozen shoulder or periarthritis shoulder is a separate disease entity and does not denote shoulder stiffness due to subacromial pathology. The cause for this common problem is poorly understood but may be multifactorial. Diabetes mellitus, trauma, cervical syndromes, autoimmune processes, pancoast tumor, thyroid disorders, Parkinson disease, head injuries, and myocardial infarction have all been associated with the development of adhesive capsulitis.

■ SYMPTOMS

Patients between 40 and 70 years of age are commonly affected. Early symptoms consist of night pain and sleeping difficulties. As the disease progresses, the predominant symptoms are increasing limitation of glenohumeral motion and pain with overhead arm use or when reaching behind the back (e.g., to tie an apron). With passage of time, these movements cause excruciating pain and eventually cannot be performed at all. The natural history consists of three phases:
1. *Phase I (pain phase)*: Duration: 2-9 months. The patient complains of acute pain that worsens at night and interferes with sleep. The predominant symptoms are pain and increasing limitation of motion (freezing phase).
2. *Phase II (frozen phase)*: Duration: 4-12 months. Symptoms consist of pain with increasing motion loss and secondary muscular atrophy.
3. *Phase III (thawing phase)*: Duration: 6-9 months. This phase is characterized by a gradual return of motion.

■ CLINICAL DIAGNOSIS

The physical findings are stage-dependent. Patients typically present with a very painful shoulder that initially retains some motion but becomes increasingly stiff. The restriction involves both active and passive shoulder movements.

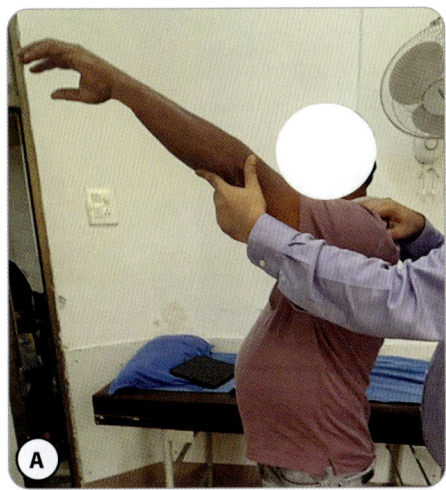
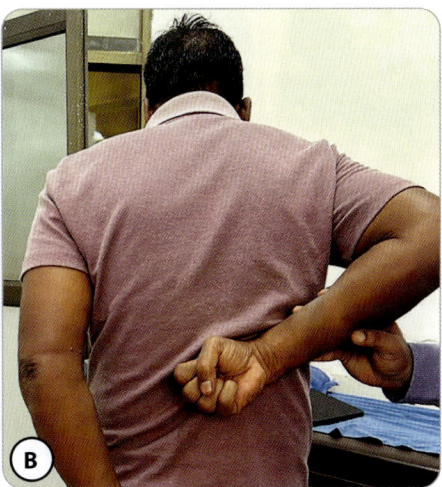
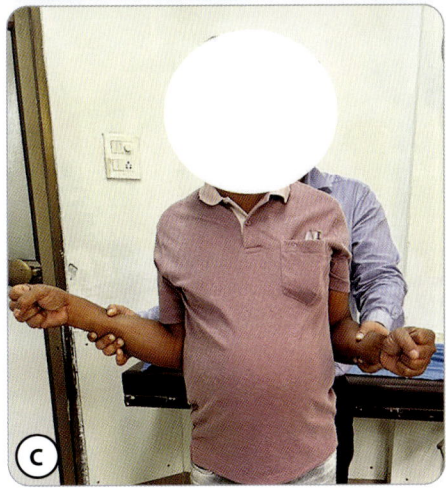

FIGS. 1A TO C: Restricted shoulder movements. (A) Forward elevation; (B) Internal rotation; and (C) External rotation.

The limitation of motion, which particularly affects rotation and abduction, is documented by clinical examination **(Figs. 1A to C)**.

Frozen shoulder requires differentiation from other conditions that cause restriction of shoulder motion: rotator cuff tears, old shoulder dislocations, calcifying rotator cuff tendinitis, and osteoarthritis. Differentiation from subacromial syndrome is also required.

■ RADIOGRAPHS, MAGNETIC RESONANCE IMAGING, AND ULTRASOUND

Radiographic and ultrasound findings in frozen shoulders are usually normal. Local osteopenia is sometimes noted. Ultrasound (USG) may show rotator interval thickening. Magnetic resonance imaging (MRI) will show inferior glenohumeral ligament (IGHL) thickening in the axillary pouch and inflammation in the rotator interval **(Figs. 2A and B)**.

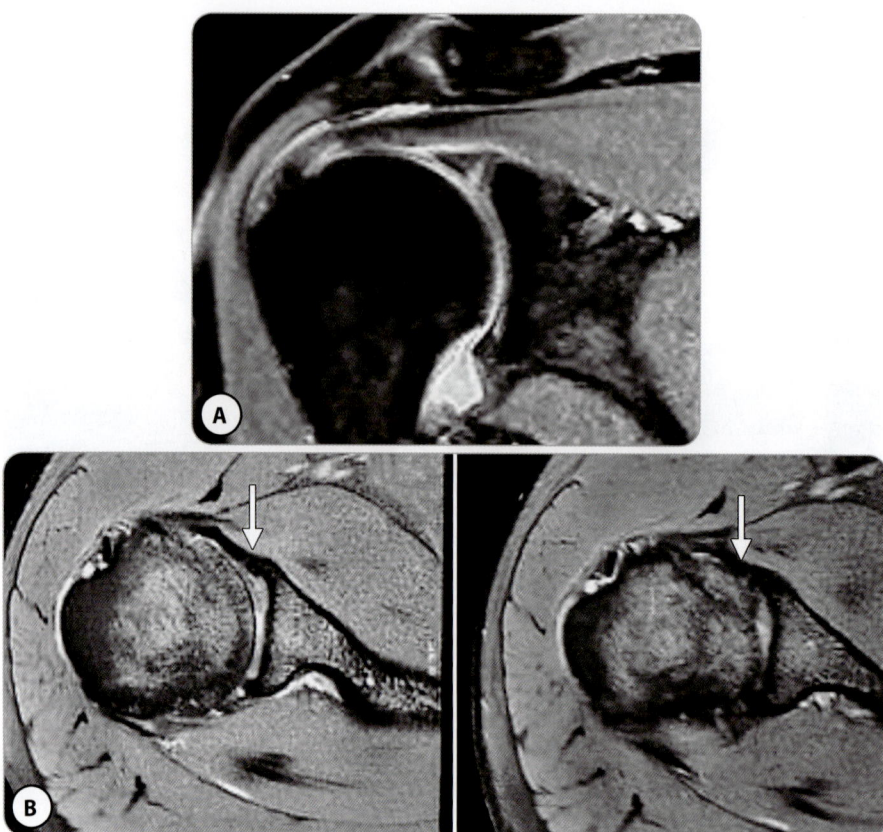

FIGS. 2A AND B: (A) MRI showing inflamed joint, and (B) MRI showing thickened IGHL (white arrows).

(IGHL: inferior glenohumeral ligament; MRI: magnetic resonance imaging)

■ ARTHROSCOPIC FINDINGS

The arthroscopic findings vary with the stage of the disease. Phase I is characterized by massive synovial hypertrophy and phase II by a marked decrease in joint volume (capsular contraction), obliteration of the axillary recess by adhesions, and marked induration of the joint capsule **(Figs. 3A and B)**.

■ THERAPEUTIC MANAGEMENT

Reports on the natural history of this disease are contradictory. Several years ago, frozen shoulder was thought to be a self-limiting disease in which complete recovery of shoulder function occurred in 1–2 years on average. Long-term studies have shown, however, that recovery of motion can be greatly prolonged and that significant motion deficits may persist.

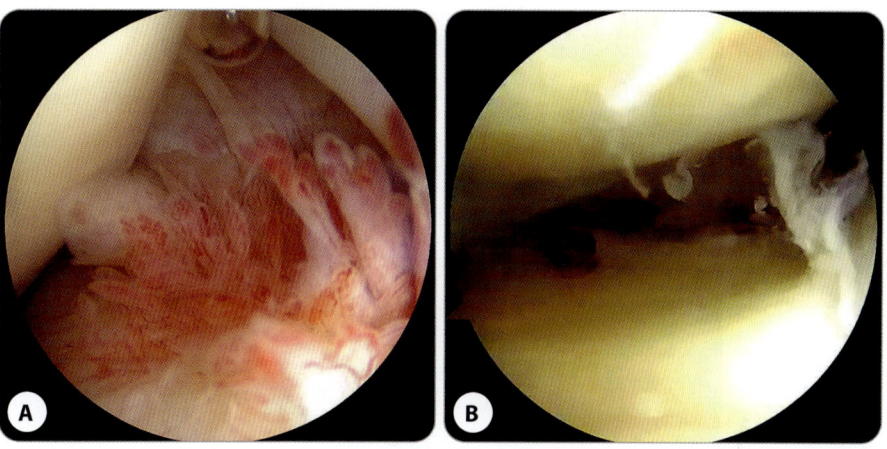

FIGS. 3A AND B: (A) Inflamed rotator interval, and (B) Tight joint.

CONSERVATIVE TREATMENT

Primary treatment is symptomatic, consisting of nonsteroidal anti-inflammatory agents and analgesic medications. Sedatives and calcitonin are beneficial in some cases. Intra-articular corticosteroid injections combined with physical therapy may also be tried. The goal of physical therapy is to improve pain and motion by stretching the muscles and capsule.

Manipulation under anesthesia: The patient's arm is grasped just below the elbow, and the other hand is placed in the axilla to obtain the shortest possible lever arm. The arm is now passively anteverted at the shoulder joint. The hand in the axilla can feel a decrease in soft tissue resistance accompanied by snapping and tearing sounds, usually between 80 and 120°. Next, the arm is gently externally rotated and simultaneously abducted to 90°.

OPERATIVE TECHNIQUE

Arthroscope portal: Sheath insertion can be difficult in a frozen shoulder due to the restricted joint play and indurated capsule. The operation should be reserved for experienced surgeons, therefore. When the sheath is intra-articular, the joint is distended with fluid. A normal degree of expansion is not obtained because of the contracted capsule. However, the fluid distention itself provides a therapeutic effect by stretching the capsule. At times, it may be necessary to do a gentle manipulation after anesthesia to facilitate easier entry into the shoulder joint.

Instrument portal: Given the frequently tight confines in a frozen shoulder joint, particular care must be exercised when creating the anterior inferior instrument portal. The Wissinger rod technique should be used.

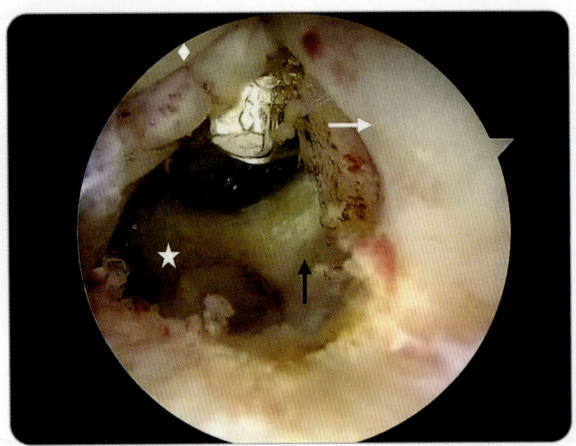

FIG. 4: Completed rotator interval release. Coracoid process (star), conjoint tendon (black arrow), long head biceps tendon (white arrow), and humeral head (diamond).

Partial synovectomy and rotator interval release: It is common to find diffuse synovitis, adhesions, and contracted tissue in the anterior part of the joint. In this case, a partial synovectomy should be performed, and adhesive bands should be removed as required. Rotator interval release is then done using an electrocautery **(Fig. 4)**.

Capsular release: 270° anterior and posterior capsular release is done using an electrocautery. As the axillary nerve is in close proximity to the glenoid at the 6 o'clock position, the capsulotomy here is performed with an arthroscopy scissors to avoid injury to the axillary nerve **(Figs. 5A to C)**.

Subacromial bursectomy: The arthroscope is advanced into the subacromial space, which is cleared of scar tissue and adhesions. If possible, subacromial decompression is not performed. In cases with a curved or a hooked acromion, an acromioplasty is also performed.

Arthroscopic inspection: The final condition of the joint is evaluated arthroscopically. Local bleeding sites are controlled with electrocautery.

Steroid injection: An intra-articular corticosteroid injection can be administered under arthroscopic control to reduce the synovitis.

■ POSTOPERATIVE CARE

An intensive exercise program is essential and should include manual therapy to improve joint mobility (distraction, translation, and separation exercises). Plexus anesthesia (Winnie block) is helpful in the postoperative period. Continuous passive motion is started on the first postoperative day. A cold therapy pad (e.g., Polar Care) can be used to reduce pain and swelling.

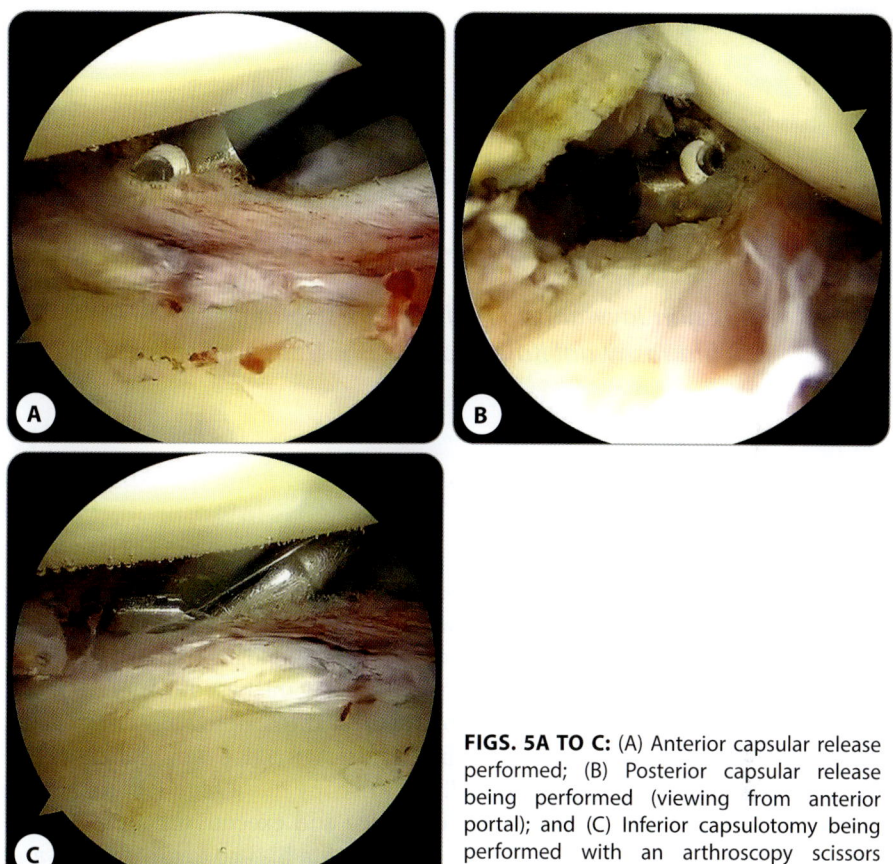

FIGS. 5A TO C: (A) Anterior capsular release performed; (B) Posterior capsular release being performed (viewing from anterior portal); and (C) Inferior capsulotomy being performed with an arthroscopy scissors (viewing from the posterior portal).

SUGGESTED READING

1. Strobel MJ (Ed). Manual of Arthroscopic Surgery. Berlin: Springer; 2002. pp. 926-8.

CHAPTER 13

The Psychology of an Arthroscopy Surgeon

Bhushan Jaywantrao Patil, Anup Krishnan,
Sachin Yashwant Kale, Pramod Bhor, Sachiti Sachin Kale

■ INTRODUCTION

The role of an arthroscopy surgeon extends far beyond the technical expertise of performing minimally invasive procedures. While skill in handling tools and instruments during surgery is crucial, the psychological landscape of an arthroscopy surgeon is equally significant in ensuring the best outcomes.

This chapter delves into the psychology of the arthroscopic surgeon, focusing on several essential traits that shape the mindset, practice, and patient interaction in this high-stakes medical field. Arthroscopy has a high learning curve and needs a large number of cases to expertise and execute the surgical procedures. Like an artist, the surgeon has to keep aside his ego to understand and learn new techniques.

■ ARTHROSCOPY SURGEON LIKE AN EVENT MANAGER

Performing arthroscopic surgery is like event management. The surgeon has to perform multiple tasks in the operation theater (OT). He must assure all the preoperative formalities, set of equipment, necessary instruments, implants, and assure that disposables have been arranged. He has to be attentive throughout the surgical procedure.

While performing the surgery, the surgeon has to maneuver arthroscope in different portals with knee and shoulder in different positions, use shaver/radio frequency (RF) footswitch, use different instruments, and keep a watch on normal saline.

Usually, the shaver system which may give trouble to the surgeon. I remember many occasions where the shaver handpiece/machine broke down during the procedure and the surgeon had to arrange the alternative system.

More than a surgical procedure, arranging the arthroscopy set, instruments, and implants and other equipment in OT is a more tedious job for the surgeon.

So, the arthroscopy surgeon prefers to work with a team and distribute the responsibilities to his assistants.

We can enjoy our work only if we are stress free and execute the surgical procedure.

■ PATIENCE: SHORT TERM AND LONG TERM

Arthroscopy is a technically difficult procedure, and we need to have patience while performing the surgery as well as during the entire journey as an arthroscopist.

We may struggle even for minor procedures like meniscectomy in an early phase. I have seen surgeons struggling and taking more than an hour to remove the bucket handle tear of the meniscus. But that is the learning phase, and every surgeon goes through the same phase.

While operating, the most important thing is to prevent iatrogenic damage to the normal structures, e.g., cartilage. Cartilage scuffing is the permanent damage and may cause recurrent effusion and persistence of pain postoperatively.

We need equally good assistants to facilitate good vision of the structures, especially the posterior horn of the medial meniscus.

While learning the arthroscopic procedures, the surgeon may go through the phases of frustration. Unavoidable iatrogenic damage, difficult operative scenario, difficulty in orientation while performing the surgery especially rotator cuff repair or meniscus repair.

I remember my seniors instructing us not to perform major procedures unless well oriented with joint anatomy and enough hands on with minor procedures. Assisting an adequate number of cases is essential before starting the arthroscopy practice.

■ LEARNING CURVE

Though it has a high learning curve **(Fig. 1)**, it has been reduced nowadays by educational/academic activities/hands on workshops organized all over with established arthroscopy surgeons involved as a faculty.

In the learning process, we learn: What to do? then How to do?

To understand how to do, we must attend surgeries with the expert surgeon and try to follow in his footsteps. Hands-on workshops are the best way to learn in an early phase of the arthroscopy career.

Fortunately, in recent years, there are many conferences/workshops and online clinical activities happening which help us to learn advances in the field and upgrade ourselves.

To execute the surgical procedure, all the necessary steps of the surgery should be understood and revised by the operating surgeon.

In sports psychology, there is a technique known as "visualization". It has shown great benefits to the sports people and commonly followed by the professional athletes.

I follow and advise my juniors to use this technique. In this visualization technique, the surgeon imagines that he is performing the arthroscopic surgery with all the minute details and necessary steps till the end. These surgical steps have to be revised and visualized multiple times in mind. It trains our brain and helps to build our confidence and reduce anxiety while performing the surgery.

After every surgical procedure, the surgeon should understand the mistakes made and the difficulties faced. Accepting the mistakes and errors is the most essential part of the learning **(Fig. 2)**.

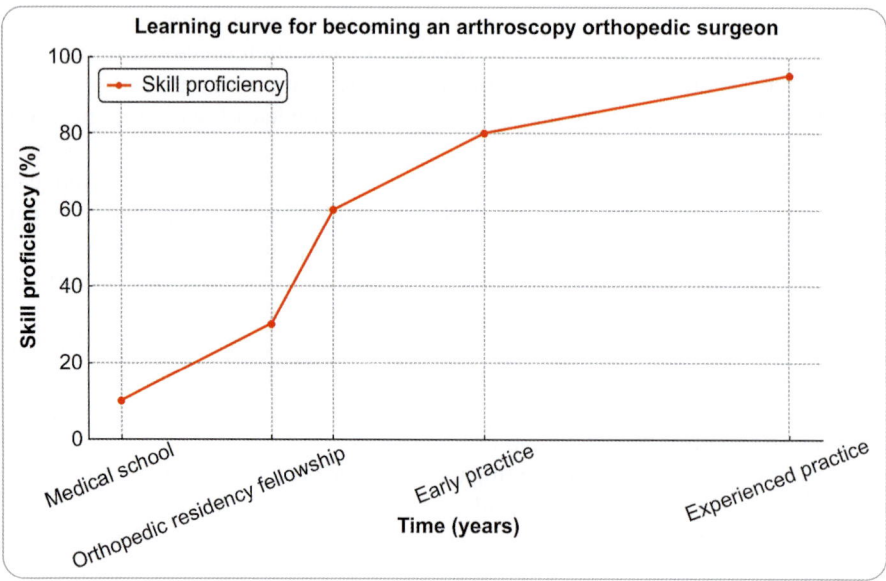

FIG. 1: Arthroscopy being a technically demanding procedure has a high learning curve.

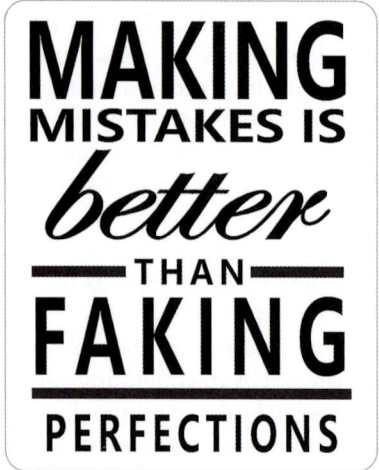

FIG. 2: Motivational image.

Then one should discuss and learn with colleagues/seniors personally or during the conferences/workshops. Effective learning is possible during the hands-on workshops and while performing the live surgery.

Postoperative complications should be evaluated thoroughly by the operating surgeon to understand the exact cause.

It is said that "we learn when we make a mistake". Making a mistake is not a crime but not learning through it may be.

PATIENT SELECTION: THE KEY TO SUCCESS

- Understanding the history, clinical evaluation, and clinical correlation is the most crucial part in decision making.
- We should never rely only on MRI for the decision making. Clinical correlation is the most important for decision making.
- As a treating doctor, we should be able to read the X-ray/MRI films and not rely on the reports.
- The surgeon should be clear with his decision for the surgery.

Simple formula is good indication, good execution, and good outcome.

PROPER PREOPERATIVE COUNSELING: SETTING REALISTIC EXPECTATIONS

Understanding the psychology of the patient is another fundamental aspect of an arthroscopy surgeon's practice.

Counseling the patient before the surgery is important aspect as the patient has to undergo rehabilitation program to achieve good result.

Patient has to be explained that the magical result may not be possible even after the well-executed surgical procedure.

Especially after rotator cuff repair the recovery and rehabilitation is slowly progressive, and the final outcome may take up to 1 year. Hence, the patient needs to follow-up till then.

Selecting the right patient for the right procedure involves assessing not only the physical capacity of the patient but also his psychological readiness for surgery and his demands in routine and professional life.

In many cases, especially an elite sports person may be driven by unrealistic expectations and early return to sports which may not be possible, and he has to be counseled before the surgery.

Most nonsports people, especially female patients are not motivated to undergo exercise programs and rehabilitation on the contrary the sports person has high motivational quotient but high demands and unrealistic early return to sports expectations.

Preoperative counseling serves several purposes—it educates the patient, sets realistic expectations, reduces anxiety, and builds trust.

The psychological benefits of proper counseling cannot be overstated. Patients who feel informed and involved in the decision-making process are more likely to experience reduced anxiety and increased satisfaction with their treatment, regardless of the outcome.

■ READINESS TO LEARN NEW TECHNIQUES: STAYING UPDATED IN A DYNAMIC FIELD

As I mentioned earlier, we need to have an approach like an artist.

We need to learn and adapt to the newer techniques and advances in the field every now then.

At the same time, we need to stick to the principles and ideal indications for the particular procedure.

Performing any technique for the unindicated reason may create complications and unnecessary stressful situations for the surgeon.

Selecting the patient for the meniscus repair/rotator cuff repair is crucial. In early stages of the career, the patient selection is an important factor.

While operating, we need to be sure about the chances of tissue healing if repair is performed. Ideally, indicated procedure will give a good result but when in doubt, we should not perform the procedure. Because if it does not work, the patient may need a second operation and it is a very stressful situation for both.

Learning new techniques often means stepping out of one's comfort zone, which can be psychologically daunting but unless we face the situation we may not learn.

When performing new procedures, it is always better to work as a team. Inviting an experienced surgeon/colleague to perform/assist the surgical procedure is always a better approach and could be a great learning experience.

■ TRANSPARENT RELATIONSHIP WITH PATIENTS: BUILDING TRUST

A transparent, honest relationship between surgeon and patient is foundational to the success of any surgical procedure. We should possibly try to explain every point mentioned on the procedure consent.

Showing photographs/video of the previously performed successful cases helps to gain patient confidence and ease in convincing him for surgery.

Patients who trust their surgeon are more likely to adhere to preoperative and postoperative instructions, experience less anxiety, and report greater satisfaction with their care.

Informing details of the surgical procedure helps to gain the patient's confidence and easy to explain the postoperative protocol especially after the meniscus repair and rotator cuff repair.

In case of a complication, the patient has to be informed of the exact cause and the further management. In this situation, listening to the patient, giving adequate time to him and gradually explaining to him the exact cause may be helpful to gain his confidence and the further management.

POSTOPERATIVE REHABILITATION

Preoperative clear communication with both the patient and their family about the rehabilitation process is crucial. We need to explain the timeline for recovery and the importance of the rehabilitation program.

Usually, patients have misconception about the word "physiotherapy".

We need to explain to them that exercise program is the most important factor for the outcome and rarely any modalities are required. Most of the surgeons prefer to explain this exercise program on their own to prevent undue overtraining and complications.

First 2 months postoperatively, it is important to keep weekly follow-ups and assess pain/discomfort and functional improvement. Exercise programs should be modified and designed accordingly.

If required, the patient has to be referred to the experienced therapist who understands and works in coordination with the operating surgeon.

Patients with a positive approach have a faster recovery and early functional return.

Postoperatively many patients, especially homemaker ladies, return to work as soon as they feel better despite surgeons' advice. In this situation, they come back to us with an increase in pain and joint swelling.

As a surgeon, we should not be mechanical in managing the patient. Being emotionally supportive is more important than performing the surgery technically correctly.

Being empathetic toward the patient benefits us in both scenarios—whether achieving a successful outcome or managing postoperative complications. If there is a good outcome, naturally he will appreciate and spread good opinion about the surgeon and in case of complication, it is much easier to discuss and convince about the further management plan.

In a clinical practice, we face different patient personalities. From patients who are very obedient and get all the past records and keep regular follow-up to some patients who have extremely casual approach and irregular follow-up. While managing any of these patients, we need to tackle the situation without losing our temper and insist on the factors which are necessary for the functional outcome.

CONCLUSION: THE MINDSET OF A SUCCESSFUL ARTHROSCOPIC SURGEON

The psychology of an arthroscopic surgeon is multifaceted, from being clinically relevant, specific in treatment planning, technically perfect surgeon, good counselor, and aware of the rehabilitation program to achieve good functional outcome.

By cultivating these psychological traits, an arthroscopy surgeon can provide exceptional care, continuously improve his skills, and build lasting relationships

with his patients, ultimately contributing to the advancement of their field and the well-being of those they serve.
- *The mental and emotional challenges of an orthopedic surgeon*: A review" Examines the psychological stressors faced by orthopedic surgeons, including arthroscopists.
- "*Surgeon resilience and burnout*: How to stay mentally tough in a high-stakes profession"—journal of surgical education discusses burnout, coping strategies, and maintaining mental well-being.
- "*Decision making in arthroscopy*: A cognitive perspective"—american journal of sports medicine analyzes cognitive load, surgical decision-making, and psychological preparedness in arthroscopy

■ SUGGESTED READINGS

1. Books on Surgical Psychology and Performance:
    - "The Mental Side of Surgery: An Essential Guide for Every Surgeon" – Kevin R Loughlin Covers mental preparedness, stress management, and decision-making for surgeons.
    - "Peak: Secrets from the New Science of Expertise" – Anders Ericsson and Robert Pool Explores deliberate practice and skill acquisition, relevant to arthroscopic precision.
    - "Thinking, Fast and Slow" – Daniel Kahneman
2. Articles on Surgical Decision-Making and Mental Resilience:
    - "Cognitive and Psychomotor Skills in Arthroscopic Surgery: The Role of Training and Simulation" – Journal of Bone and Joint Surgery
    - "Mental Toughness in Surgeons: Psychological Factors Influencing Performance in the Operating Room" – Annals of Surgery
    - "Decision-Making Under Uncertainty in Surgery" – British Journal of Surgery
3. Research on Stress and Burnout in Surgeons:
    - "Burnout Among Orthopedic Surgeons: Causes, Consequences, and Coping Strategies" – Journal of Orthopaedic Trauma

CHAPTER 14

Rehabilitation in Knee Ligament Arthroscopic Surgeries

Sagar Subhash Deshpande, Prerna Pradeep Ghodke, Sachin Yashwant Kale

■ INTRODUCTION

Knee ligament injuries are common in sports populations, military training, and high-demand professionals. The best indication for ligament surgery is a clinical assessment with a risk of reinjury. Arthroscopic surgery is used to repair/reconstruct the severe form of knee ligament injury because it is less intrusive and speeds up recovery. For healthy, active patients, full recovery from ligament surgeries typically takes 6–9 months. A long-term rehabilitation provides good joint stability and a return to preinjury activity levels. It is crucial to perform frequent quadriceps exercises by straightening the knee and lifting the leg with the knee as straight as possible because there is a tendency for muscle wasting to happen rather quickly if exercises are not done. Thus, rehabilitation is designed based on the graft used and the functional demands of the patients. Determining whether to start open kinetic chain (OKC) exercises is crucial to rehabilitating these injuries. For recovery following reconstruction surgeries, closed kinetic chain (CKC) exercises have often been recommended over OKC exercises. This preference stemmed from the idea that, in comparison to CKC exercises, OKC exercises could place greater strain on the reconstructed anterior cruciate ligament (ACL), increasing knee discomfort, and laxity. However, studies have shown that OKC exercises showed greater quadriceps strength during the return to activity period whether in a conservative or surgically managed ACL. If started in the second or sixth postoperative week, there is consistent evidence that OKC training and CKC exercise can considerably increase quadriceps strength compared to CKC exercise alone. This suggests that both OKC and CKC exercises contribute to the recovery after ligament surgeries. However, OKC exercises within a limited range of motion (ROM) (45–90°) in the initial stages of rehabilitation could be a safer option. Since OKC exercises increase graft tension, they must be used carefully starting 4 weeks after anterior cruciate ligament reconstruction (ACLR). The efficient functioning of the knee extensor mechanism is critical to overcome the injury. **Table 1** summarizes the goals and interventions of the rehabilitation in each phase.

TABLE 1: Long-term rehabilitation of knee ligament arthroscopic surgeries.

Rehabilitation protocol		Phase 1 Immediate postoperative phase	Phase 2 Intermediate postoperative phase	Phase 3 Late postoperative phase	Phase 4 Return to activity/function phase	Phase 5 Return to recreational activity/sports phase
Conditions	Duration	0–2 weeks	3–6 weeks	6–9 weeks	9–12 weeks	12 weeks to 5 months
• Anterior cruciate ligament (ACL) reconstruction • Meniscus repair • Meniscectomy • ACL, MCL, MM (terrible triad injury)	Common goals	• Patient counseling • Protection of the graft • Minimize pain and swelling • Prevent extension lag • Prevent arthrogenic muscle inhibition • Adequate quadriceps contraction • Prevent muscle tightness • Initiate gait training with a walking aid • Prevent immediate postoperative complications	• Continue graft protection • Improve neuromuscular control • Improve muscle flexibility • Improve quadriceps and hamstring strength • Improve knee proprioception • Improve joint stability • Initiate open-chain exercises • Progress with gait training	• Maintain muscle flexibility • Improve motor control • Improve proprioception and balance • Maintain joint stability • Improve quadriceps and hamstring strength	• Maintain knee proprioception • Improve muscle strength and endurance • Improve balance and coordination • Improve aerobic fitness • Improve neuromuscular control	• Maintain full ROM • Increase aerobic fitness • Achieve maximum muscle strength and endurance • Improve sports-specific explosive power • Improve multidirectional balance and proprioception • Improve neuromuscular control • Improve load absorption • Skill-specific training **(Fig. 1)** • Achieve sports-specific fatigue • Sports psychology and nutritional counseling

Continued

Continued

Rehabilitation protocol		Phase 1 Immediate postoperative phase	Phase 2 Intermediate postoperative phase	Phase 3 Late postoperative phase	Phase 4 Return to activity/function phase	Phase 5 Return to recreational activity/sports phase
Conditions	Duration	0–2 weeks	3–6 weeks	6–9 weeks	9–12 weeks	12 weeks to 5 months
ACL reconstruction	Specific goals (ROM, bracing, and weight-bearing status)	• Improve knee ROM (0–90°) • Long knee brace (first week) • Protective weightbearing with walking aid	• Maintain knee ROM (0–110°) • Hinged knee brace • Full weightbearing as tolerated with/without a walking aid • Encourage heel-to-toe gait	• Maintain knee ROM (0–125°) • Full weight bearing • Hinged knee brace • Encourage heel-to-toe gait	• Maintain knee ROM (0–135°) • Neoprene sleeve • Full weight-bearing	• Maintain full ROM at the knee • Neoprene sleeve • Full weightbearing
Meniscus repair		• Improve knee ROM (0–70°) • Long knee brace • Partial weightbearing	• Improve knee ROM (0–90°) • Hinged knee brace • Partial weightbearing	• Improve knee ROM (0–120°) • Hinged knee brace • Partial weightbearing to full weightbearing as tolerated	• Improve knee ROM (0–135°) • Neoprene sleeve • Full weight-bearing	• Maintain full ROM at the knee • Neoprene sleeve • Full weightbearing
Meniscectomy		• Improve knee ROM (0–90°) • Long knee brace (first week) • Weightbearing as tolerated with crutches	• Improve knee ROM (0–120°) • Hinged knee brace • Full weightbearing	• Improve knee ROM (0–135°) • Hinged knee brace • Full weightbearing	• Maintain full ROM at the knee • Neoprene sleeve • Full weight-bearing	• Maintain full ROM at the knee • Neoprene sleeve • Full weightbearing

Continued

Rehabilitation protocol		Phase 1 Immediate postoperative phase	Phase 2 Intermediate postoperative phase	Phase 3 Late postoperative phase	Phase 4 Return to activity/function phase	Phase 5 Return to recreational activity/sports phase
Conditions	Duration	0–2 weeks	3–6 weeks	6–9 weeks	9–12 weeks	12 weeks to 5 months
ACL, MCL, and MM/LM (terrible triad injury)	Intervention	• Improve knee ROM (<90°) • Long knee brace • Non-weightbearing *Mobility:* • Ankle pumps • Elevation and compression for swelling reduction • Passive patellafemoral mobilization • Passive tibiofemoral mobilization • Supine heel slides and wall slides • Supine gastrocnemius/soleus stretch • Passive ROM (0–90°) • Passive VMO activation	• Improve knee ROM (0–90°) • Hinged knee brace • Partial weightbearing *Mobility:* Continue phase 1 exercises • Active assisted prone hamstring curls • Initiate gentle hamstring stretch • Posterior capsule stretch • Prone quadriceps stretch • Thomas stretch for iliopsoas • TFL and IT band stretch **(Fig. 2)** • Active VMO activation • Standing hamstring curls after 4 weeks	• Improve knee ROM (0–125°) • Hinged knee brace • Partial to full weightbearing *Mobility:* Continue phase 1 and 2 exercises • Initiate forward and lateral lunges • Standing quadriceps stretch • IT band stretch/foam roller • Static cycling with resistance • Supine unilateral bridging • Wall squats (0–90°) • Step-up exercises (up to 8 inches) **(Fig. 3)** • Obstacle walking	• Maintain full ROM at the knee • Neoprene sleeve • Full weightbearing *Mobility:* • Warm up with 10 minutes of cycling • Balance and proprioception training on an unstable surface **(Fig. 4)** • Step-ups and lateral step-ups (up to 12 inches) • Plyometric training • Retrograde walking on a treadmill	• Maintain full ROM at the knee • Neoprene sleeve • Full weightbearing *Mobility:* • Warm up with 10–20 minutes of cycling or running • Single-leg balance on an unstable surface **(Fig. 5)** • Plyometric training • Step-ups and lateral step-ups (up to 18–20 inches) • Sports-specific cardiovascular training • Retrograde treadmill walking • Reduce ground contact time

Continued

Continued

Rehabilitation protocol

Conditions	Duration	Phase 1 Immediate postoperative phase 0–2 weeks	Phase 2 Intermediate postoperative phase 3–6 weeks	Phase 3 Late postoperative phase 6–9 weeks	Phase 4 Return to activity/function phase 9–12 weeks	Phase 5 Return to recreational activity/sports phase 12 weeks to 5 months
		• *Hip mobility exercises:* SLR and hip abduction • *Soft tissue manipulation* to quadriceps, hamstrings, and calf • *Prone hangs* if extension lag is present • *Sit-to-stand transfer training* *Strengthening:* • Static quadriceps sets • *Core strengthening exercises:* TA activation • *Hip strengthening:* Static gluteal sets and short hip flexor activation	• Retrograde walking • Static cycling without resistance • Initiate step-up, step-down, lateral step-up exercises (2–4 inches step) **(Fig. 6)** *Strengthening:* • Supine bridging • Hip clamshell exercise • Hip abductor strengthening • Progression of TA activation • Multiple angle isometrics to quadriceps in sitting • Mini wall squats (0–45°) **(Fig. 7)** • Heel raises with support	*Strengthening:* • Seated leg extension (90–45°) with weights **(Fig. 8)** • Strengthening of quadriceps and hamstrings • Leg press exercise (45° of knee flexion –0°) • Resisted hamstring curls • Recumbent bicycling with mild resistance • Core strengthening • Balance training on an unstable surface • Progress to single-leg balance training • Balance with perturbation	*Strengthening:* • Leg press (90° of knee flexion–0°) with resistance • Body weight squats • Single leg squat • Closed chain core strengthening exercises • Agility drills **(Fig. 9)**	*Strengthening:* • Body weight squats • Deadlift • Front squats • Box jumps • Bounding • Sprinting • Hopping • Jumping with a soft landing • Agility drills • Sports-specific strengthening

Continued

Rehabilitation protocol		Phase 1 Immediate postoperative phase	Phase 2 Intermediate postoperative phase	Phase 3 Late postoperative phase	Phase 4 Return to activity/ function phase	Phase 5 Return to recreational activity/sports phase
Conditions	Duration	0–2 weeks	3–6 weeks	6–9 weeks	9–12 weeks	12 weeks to 5 months
	Modality	• Cryotherapy for 15–20 minutes (Fig. 10) • Neuromuscular electrical stimulation for muscle contraction • Continuous passive movement (0–70°) • Upper extremity strengthening	• Toes raise with support • Balance training with a bilateral stance • Biofeedback/ electrical stimulation • Aquatic therapy • Dry needling • Cupping therapy • Matrix rhythm therapy (Fig. 11)	• Blood flow restriction training • Aquatic therapy	• Blood flow restriction training	
Prerequisites for progression		• Minimal pain and swelling • No extension lag • Knee ROM 90° • Absence of antalgic gait • SLR without extension lag	• No pain and swelling • Knee ROM 110° • Quadriceps strength >50% of the uninvolved side • Normal gait pattern • Normal patella mobility • Full weightbearing without walking aid	• No pain or signs of active inflammation • Knee ROM up to 120–130° • Quadriceps and hamstring strength >70% of the uninvolved side • Able to jog or run • No compensation in squat	• No pain • Full ROM at the knee • Hop test >90% • Quadriceps strength 90% of the uninvolved side • Able to run comfortably	

Continued

Rehabilitation protocol		Phase 1 Immediate postoperative phase	Phase 2 Intermediate postoperative phase	Phase 3 Late postoperative phase	Phase 4 Return to activity/function phase	Phase 5 Return to recreational activity/sports phase
Conditions	Duration	0–2 weeks	3–6 weeks	6–9 weeks	9–12 weeks	12 weeks to 5 months
				• Hop test >80% • Unilateral stance for 20–30 seconds • Ascent and descent of stairs without compensation		

Note: The rehabilitation may change as per the graft used and as directed by the surgeon.

General precautions:
- Avoid over stressing the donor graft site
- Pain and swelling will help guide the stage of tissue healing and exercise progression
- Weightbearing as tolerated
- Long knee brace should be locked in 0° extension
- Open-chain exercises can begin after 4 weeks within safe limits of ROM
- The ROM guidelines will change as per the graft used and associated injuries
- The timeline for return to sports may vary based on preinjury activity level and patient goals

(IT: iliotibial; LM: lateral meniscus; MCL: medial collateral ligament; MM: medial meniscus; ROM: range of motion; SLR: straight leg raise; TA: transverse abdominis; TFL: tensor fascia lata; VMO: vastus medialis obliquus)

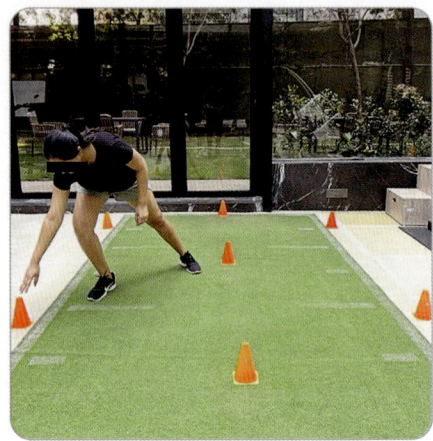

FIG. 1: Knee agility and cutting sports-specific drills.

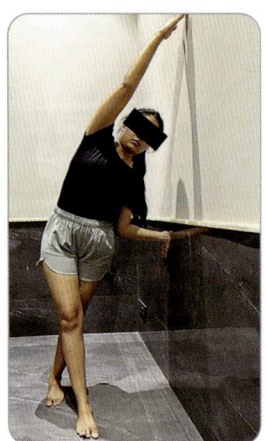

FIG. 2: Tensor fascia latae stretch.

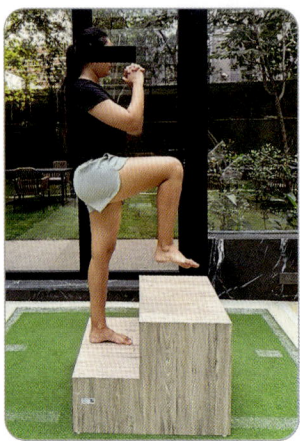

FIG. 3: Step-up exercise.

CHAPTER 14: Rehabilitation in Knee Ligament Arthroscopic Surgeries

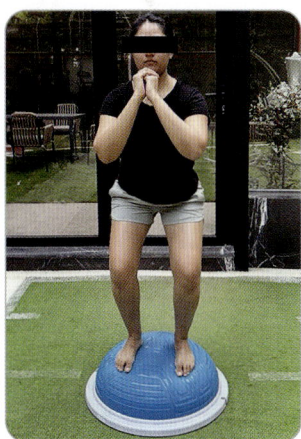

FIG. 4: Knee proprioception training.

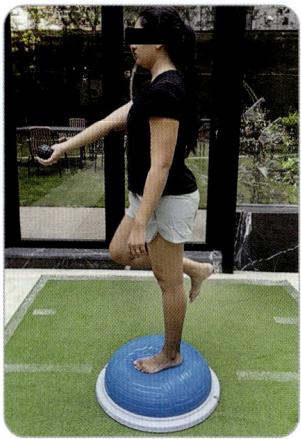

FIG. 5: Single leg balance training.

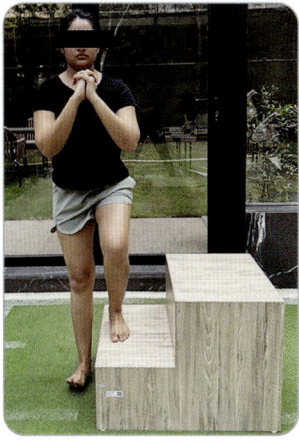

FIG. 6: Lateral step ups.

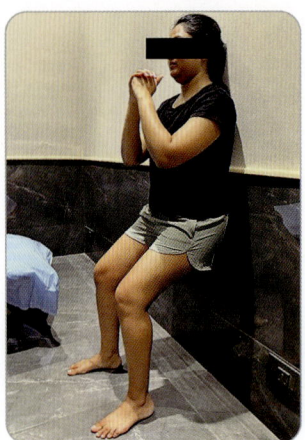

FIG. 7: Mini wall squats.

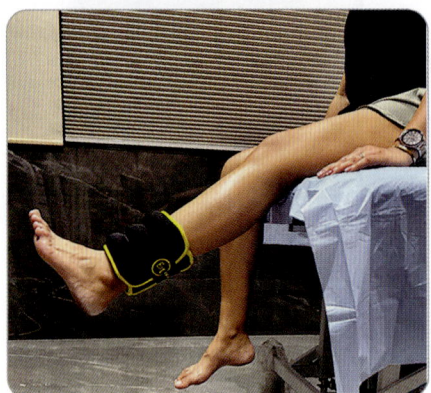

FIG. 8: Dynamic quadriceps strengthening.

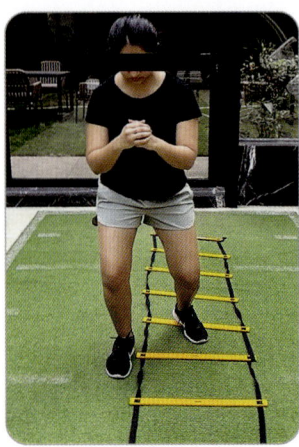

FIG. 9: Agility ladder drills.

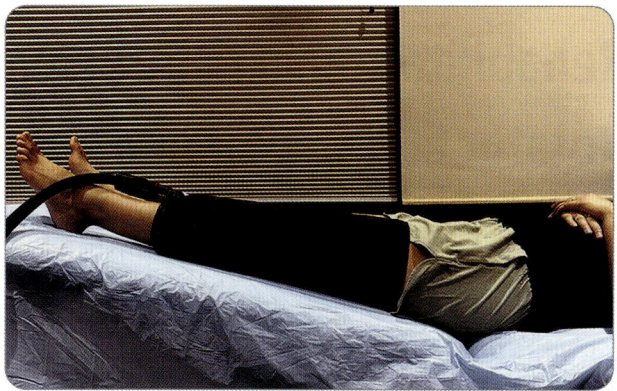

FIG. 10: Cryocompression therapy with limb elevation.

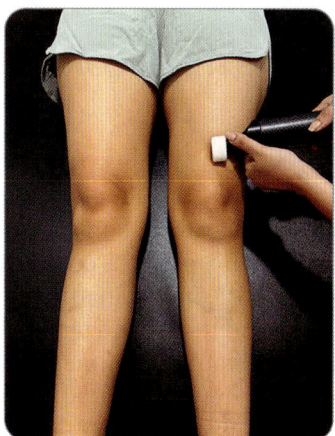

FIG. 11: Matrix rhythm therapy.

■ SUGGESTED READINGS

1. Sood M, Kulshrestha V, Kumar S, Kumar P, Amaravati RS, Singh S. Trends and beliefs in ACL reconstruction surgery: Indian perspectives. J Clin Orthop Trauma. 2023;39:102148.
2. Ariel de Lima D, Helito CP, Lima FRA de, Leite JAD. Surgical indications for anterior cruciate ligament reconstruction combined with extra-articular lateral tenodesis or anterolateral ligament reconstruction. Rev Bras Ortop (English Ed). 2018;53(6):661-7.
3. Pamboris GM, Pavlou K, Paraskevopoulos E, Mohagheghi AA. Effect of open vs. closed kinetic chain exercises in ACL rehabilitation on knee joint pain, laxity, extensor muscles strength, and function: a systematic review with meta-analysis. Front Sport Act Living. 2024;6:1416690.
4. Culvenor AG, Girdwood MA, Juhl CB, Patterson BE, Haberfield MJ, Holm PM, et al. Rehabilitation after anterior cruciate ligament and meniscal injuries: a best-evidence synthesis of systematic reviews for the OPTIKNEE consensus. Br J Sports Med. 2022;56(24):1445-53.
5. Yang YP, Ma X, An H, Liu XP, An N, Ao YF. Meniscus repair with simultaneous anterior cruciate ligament reconstruction: Clinical outcomes, failure rates and subsequent processing. Chinese J Traumatol. 2022;25(1):37-44.
6. Mesnard G, Fournier G, Joseph L, Shatrov JG, Lustig S, Servien E. Does meniscal repair impact muscle strength following ACL reconstruction? SICOT-J. 2022;8:16.

CHAPTER 15

Rehabilitation in Arthroscopic Rotator Cuff Repair and Capsular Release in Frozen Shoulder

Sagar Subhash Deshpande, Prerna Pradeep Ghodke, Sachin Yashwant Kale

■ REHABILITATION IN ARTHROSCOPIC ROTATOR CUFF REPAIR

The tendons of supraspinatus, infraspinatus, subscapularis, and teres minor together form the rotator cuff (RC). The shoulder joint is the most mobile in the body owing to the dynamic stabilization these muscles provide. When the subscapularis and infraspinatus create a compressive joint reaction force in the axial plane, the deltoid and supraspinatus act as a force couple in the coronal plane, compressing the humeral head to the glenoid in abduction. This provides dynamic stabilization to the glenohumeral (GH) joint. The rotator cuff tendons under the acromion undergo repeated translation, causing tears of the RC as a result of shoulder impingement. As new blood vessels grow and the tendon-to-bone repair site continues to mature, it takes around 12 weeks for the repair site to start to have structural integrity after a RC arthroscopic procedure. Shoulder surgeons are constantly concerned about stiffness since it exacerbates shoulder discomfort and is generally uncomfortable. Although the surgery is still healing after 6 weeks, extended immobilization is not recommended due to the increased risk of stiffness. In order to reduce the possibility of harm to the healing tendon, the majority of patients are weaned off of the sling at 6 weeks and put into a motion restoration plan that includes particular restrictions on lifting and activities. Numerous etiological reasons can lead to RC tears, including tendon injury from restricted subacromial space and anatomical abnormalities, and tendon degradation. Every RC rupture is different, and physical therapists need to be mindful that every patient is different. For example, in order to prevent recurring tears, elderly patients or who have serious RC tears usually require a slower rehabilitation approach.

Younger patients or those with little tears in healthy tissues, however, might recover more quickly. Research shows that, in terms of long-term range of motion recovery, functional outcomes, and healing rate, delayed passive motion, early passive motion, and early active motion (EAM) were similar. At 1 year, flexion was decreased by strict immobilization as opposed to passive or active motion. Following the initial assessment, the main objective of treatment is to increase passive range of motion (PROM) and establish scapular stability. The main objectives of postsurgical rehabilitation are to prevent stiffness and muscle atrophy while facilitating healing of the repaired RC tendon. Numerous elements can help direct RC repair rehabilitation, which may ultimately lower failure rates and enhance results. These include prognostic factors, healing rate, range of motion, exercise progressions, and advice on returning to sports and job activities. **Table 1** emphasizes the long-term rehabilitation of RC repair for better outcomes.

▉ REHABILITATION IN ARTHROSCOPIC CAPSULAR RELEASE IN FROZEN SHOULDER

The intense and frequently debilitating pain and stiffness associated with frozen shoulder can significantly impact all aspects of daily life. This condition can severely limit mobility and functionality, profoundly affecting an individual's ability to perform routine activities. The three stages of frozen shoulder are described in literature as freezing, frozen, and thawing. While these stages are generally understood as consecutive, they can also overlap, making the path to recovery more complex and unpredictable. Phase one, or the freezing stage, typically lasts between 8 weeks and 3 months. Phase two, the frozen stage, persists for a duration ranging from 16 weeks to 1 year, while phase three, the thawing stage, may extend from 16 weeks to over 3 years.

Frozen shoulder may not represent a singular textbook condition but rather a spectrum of clinical phenotypes, each requiring a tailored treatment approach. Patients experiencing the most severe or persistent symptoms and those who fail conservative management or regress often resort to surgical release procedures. In addition to mitigating the risks associated with manipulation under anesthesia, arthroscopic capsular release has demonstrated considerable effectiveness in the treatment of frozen shoulder. Following such interventions, a structured rehabilitation program is typically advised to optimize recovery. The current literature suggests initiating physiotherapy within 48 hours of the procedure. The exercises are performed multiple times a day to avoid regression into stiffness and warm the shoulder up. The main objectives of postsurgical rehabilitation are to prevent stiffness, muscle atrophy, improve ROM to facilitate the capsular release, and help the patient return to full function in a safe and effective manner **Table 2**.

TABLE 1: Long-term rehabilitation of arthroscopic rotator cuff repair.

Rehabilitation protocol	Phase 1 Early postoperative phase	Phase 2 Late postoperative phase	Phase 3 Return to function/activity phase	Phase 4 Return to sports phase
Duration	0–6 weeks	7–14 weeks	14–18 weeks	18–26 weeks

Goals	• Patient counseling
	• Protect the integrity of the repaired tendon
	• Minimize pain and inflammation
	• Prevent muscle inhibition
	• Prevent postoperative complications
	• Initiate passive ROM exercises:
	  ○ Flexion (0–70°) as per patient's tolerance
	  ○ Abduction (0–60°)
	  ○ External rotation (0–30°) in scaption
		• Minimize postoperative stiffness
		• Improve scapular stabilization
		• Initiate passive ROM exercises: Flexion (0–120° as per patient's tolerance)
		  ○ Extension (0–30°)
		  ○ Abduction (0–90°)
		  ○ External rotation (0–45°) in scaption
		  ○ Internal rotation (0–30°) in scaption
		• Allow soft tissue inflammation to heal
		• Prevent capsular tightness
		• Maintain near full ROM at the shoulder
		• Improve dynamic stability of the shoulder
		• Improve muscle flexibility
		• Improve neuromuscular control and scapulohumeral rhythm
		• Proprioceptive and kinesthetic training
			• Maintain full ROM at the shoulder
			  ○ Flexion (0>120°)
			  ○ Extension (0–60°)
			  ○ Abduction (0>90°)
			  ○ External rotation (>70°) in scaption
			  ○ Internal rotation (0–60°) in scaption
			• Improve scapular stabilization
			• Improve dynamic stabilization of the GH joint
			• Improve muscle flexibility
			• Optimize neuromuscular control
			• Proprioceptive and kinesthetic training
			• Improve cardiorespiratory fitness
			• Gradual return to functional activities
				• Patient counseling
				• Continue closed chain scapula and shoulder muscle strengthening
				• Improve dynamic stabilization of the GH joint
				• Proprioceptive training
				• Improve sports-specific explosive strength, power, and endurance
				• Improve cardiorespiratory fitness
				• Gradual return to sports

Continued

Continued

Rehabilitation protocol	Phase 1 Early postoperative phase	Phase 2 Late postoperative phase	Phase 3 Return to function/activity phase	Phase 4 Return to sports phase
Duration	0–6 weeks	7–14 weeks	14–18 weeks	18–26 weeks
Bracing	Use shoulder sling for 4 weeks (remove only for exercises)	Discontinue the use of a brace or as directed by the surgeon	No brace	No brace
Intervention	*Mobility:* • Mobilization of GH and ST joints • Active ROM to elbow, wrist, and hand • Active ROM to the cervical spine • Early passive ROM till the patient's tolerance—flexion, abduction in scaption • Start passive ROM for internal and external rotation in scaption after 4 weeks • Passive ROM for abduction in coronal plane • Active assisted ROM for flexion, extension, and abduction after 4 weeks	*Mobility:* • Codman's exercise over a ball • Soft tissue mobilization to surrounding structures • Full passive ROM for flexion • Active ROM for flexion in supine using a wand • Initiate mild stretching of elbow and wrist • Side-lying external rotation • Prone extension • Side-lying scapula muscle activation • Lower and middle trapezius, rhomboids activation in prone • Eccentric control of rotator cuff • Improve external rotation in scaption, then progress to arm abducted to 90° • Proprioceptive neuromuscular facilitation (PNF) patterns	*Mobility:* • Progress to external rotation at 0 abduction • Stretching of shoulder, elbow, and wrist muscles • Prone extension • Prone horizontal abduction • Prone rowing exercises • Capsular stretching • Gym ball exercises on wall for dynamic stability *Strengthening:* • Closed chain shoulder strengthening in quadruped position • Lower and middle trapezius, rhomboids strengthening in prone • Strengthening uniplanar to multiplanar shoulder movements	*Mobility:* • Stretching of shoulder and pectoral girdle muscles • Lateral raises • Eccentric control of rotator cuff with internal and external rotation • Low resistance and high repetition for endurance training *Strengthening:* • Plyometric training—progress from bilateral to unilateral • Proprioceptive neuromuscular facilitation patterns • Agility drills • Throwing • Swimming

Continued

Continued

Rehabilitation protocol	Phase 1 Early postoperative phase	Phase 2 Late postoperative phase	Phase 3 Return to function/activity phase	Phase 4 Return to sports phase
Duration	0–6 weeks	7–14 weeks	14–18 weeks	18–26 weeks
	• Initiate active scapula retraction and depression exercises • Serratus anterior activation *Strengthening:* • Submaximal isometric contraction in flexion, extension, adduction, internal and external rotation • Grip strengthening exercises	• Capsular stretching • Muscle energy technique to improve ROM • Mobilization with movement to improve abduction and external rotation *Strengthening:* • Continue isometric strengthening as per the patient's tolerance • Kinetic control for scapulo-humeral rhythm and muscle activation • Biceps and triceps curl with mild resistance • Side-lying and prone scapula strengthening exercises (T-Y exercises) • Submaximal rhythmic stabilization for co-contraction • Serratus anterior strengthening • Resistance training after 10 weeks with mild resistance • Aquatic therapy for light ROM exercises	• Closed chain step-ups on upper extremities • Progress to overhead strengthening after 16 weeks • Isometric strengthening for flexion, extension, abduction, and rotations • Resisted diagonal PNF patterns • Resistance training using weights or resistance bands • Submaximal isokinetic training for rotations • Biceps and triceps curls with weights • Core strengthening • Aquatic therapy	• Maximal isokinetic training for rotations • Resistance training for shoulder with weights or resistance bands • Core strengthening exercises • Aquatic therapy

Continued

Continued

Rehabilitation protocol	Phase 1 Early postoperative phase	Phase 2 Late postoperative phase	Phase 3 Return to function/activity phase	Phase 4 Return to sports phase
Duration	0–6 weeks	7–14 weeks	14–18 weeks	18–26 weeks
Modality	• Cryotherapy for 10–15 minutes to minimize swelling • Transcutaneous electrical nerve stimulation (TENS) for postoperative pain	• Cryotherapy for 10–15 minutes to reduce swelling • Interferential current therapy (IFT) for muscle relaxation • TENS for postoperative pain • Low level LASER therapy • High-intensity LASER therapy • Matrix rhythm therapy	• High-intensity laser therapy • Biofeedback	Blood flow restriction training

Prerequisites for progression	• Minimal pain and no active signs of inflammation
	• Adherence to precautions
		• Adequate healing of surgical repair
		• Passive ROM of flexion (>70°)
		  ○ Extension (0–30°)
		  ○ Abduction (0–90°)
		  ○ External rotation (0–25°)
		• Appropriate scapula positioning
		• Shoulder strength—50–75% of the uninvolved side
		• Pain-free isometric exercises
			• No pain
			• No signs of active inflammation
			• Near full ROM without compensation
			• Appropriate scapular control
			• Pain-free activities of daily living
			• Shoulder strength—90% of the uninvolved side	

Continued

Continued

Rehabilitation protocol	Phase 1 Early postoperative phase	Phase 2 Late postoperative phase	Phase 3 Return to function/activity phase	Phase 4 Return to sports phase
Duration	0–6 weeks	7–14 weeks	14–18 weeks	18–26 weeks

Note: The rehabilitation may change as directed by the surgeon.

General precautions:
- Do not perform AROM till the suture removal or for 4 weeks
- Do not perform overhead activities in the initial phase
- Do not lift heavy weights on the involved side
- Do not weight bear on the involved side
- Avoid pushing and pulling activities
- Do not perform active ROM for internal rotation in the initial phase till pain and inflammation subside
- Avoid sudden jerky movements
- Maintain the arm in sling for 2 weeks
- Avoid excessive stretching in the initial 4–6 weeks

(GH: glenohumeral; ROM: range of motion)

TABLE 2: Long-term rehabilitation of arthroscopic capsular release in frozen shoulder.

Rehabilitation protocol	Phase 1 Early postoperative phase	Phase 2 Late postoperative phase	Phase 3 Early return to function/activity phase	Phase 4 Late return to function/activity phase	Phase 5 Return to sports phase
Duration	0–2 weeks	3–6 weeks	6–8 weeks	8–12 weeks	12 weeks +
Goals	• Patient counseling • Minimize pain and inflammation • Prevent muscle inhibition and joint stiffness • Prevent postoperative complications • Regain ROM as tolerated	• Prevent capsular tightness • Improve scapula stabilization ○ Achieve full ROM till the end of the phase • Improve muscle flexibility • Improve neuromuscular control and scapulohumeral rhythm • Gentle strengthening • Return to ADLs	• Maintain full ROM at the shoulder • Improve scapula stabilization • Improve dynamic stabilization of the GH joint (Fig. 1) • Improve muscle flexibility • Optimize neuromuscular control • Proprioceptive and kinesthetic training (Fig. 2) • Gradual return to functional activities	• Patient counseling • Continue closed chain scapula and shoulder muscle strengthening • Improve dynamic stabilization of the GH joint • Proprioceptive training • Improve sports-specific strength and endurance	• Improve sports-specific strength and endurance • Improve power and reactive strength
Bracing	• Use shoulder sling till the effect of block is worn off (>1 week if biceps tenodesis performed) • Wean gradually	No brace	No brace	No brace	No brace

Continued

Continued

Rehabilitation protocol	Phase 1 Early postoperative phase	Phase 2 Late postoperative phase	Phase 3 Early return to function/activity phase	Phase 4 Late return to function/activity phase	Phase 5 Return to sports phase
Duration	0–2 weeks	3–6 weeks	6–8 weeks	8–12 weeks	12 weeks +
Intervention	*Mobility:* • Passive ROM of shoulder till the block is in effect as tolerated (no active ROM) • Start active-assisted and active ROM of shoulder as tolerated after effect of block is completely worn off • Active ROM of scapulothoracic joint • Active ROM to elbow, wrist, and hand • Active ROM to the cervical spine • Mobilization of glenohumeral, acromioclavicular, and scapulothoracic joints • Codman/Pendulum exercises	*Mobility:* • Soft tissue mobilization to surrounding structures • Passive ROM as tolerated • Active ROM as tolerated • Mild capsular stretches • Muscle energy technique to improve ROM • Mobilization with movement to improve ROM • Aquatic therapy for light ROM exercises *Strengthening:* • Isotonic strengthening as per the patient's tolerance in available ROM	*Mobility:* • Active ROM ActiveROMexercises for glenohumeral joint • Capsular stretching • Gym ball exercises on wall for dynamic stability *Strengthening:* • Strengthening uniplanar to multiplanar shoulder movements • Resisted diagonal proprioceptive neuromuscular facilitation (PNF) patterns **(Figs. 3A and B)** • Resistance training of rotator cuff muscles using weights or resistance bands	*Mobility:* • Full active ROM for maintenance • Stretching of shoulder and pectoral girdle muscles • Capsular stretches • Low resistance and high repetition for endurance training *Strengthening:* • Proprioceptive neuromuscular facilitation patterns • Progress to unilateral closed chain shoulder strengthening • Agility drills • Maximal isokinetic training for rotations	*Mobility:* • Full active ROM for maintenance • Stretching of shoulder and pectoral girdle muscles • Capsular stretches • Low resistance and high repetition for endurance training *Strengthening:* • Progress maximal strength training • Plyometric training—progress from bilateral to unilateral gradually • Throwing drills

Continued

Continued

Rehabilitation protocol	Phase 1 Early postoperative phase	Phase 2 Late postoperative phase	Phase 3 Early return to function/activity phase	Phase 4 Late return to function/activity phase	Phase 5 Return to sports phase
Duration	0–2 weeks	3–6 weeks	6–8 weeks	8–12 weeks	12 weeks +
	Muscle activation: • Submaximal isometric contraction of rotator cuff muscles • Grip strengthening exercises	• Biceps and triceps curl with mild resistance • Side-lying and prone scapula strengthening exercises (T-I-Y exercises) **(Figs. 4A to D)** • Submaximal rhythmic stabilization for co-contraction • Kinetic control for scapulohumeral rhythm and muscle activation • Serratus anterior strengthening **(Fig. 5)**	• Gradually progress to bilateral closed chain shoulder strengthening in quadruped position • Submaximal isokinetic training for rotations • Aquatic therapy for strengthening • Elbow and wrist strengthening	• Resistance training for shoulder with weights or resistance bands • Core strengthening exercises	
Modality	• Transcutaneous electrical nerve stimulation (TENS) in case of postoperative pain • Low level LASER therapy/high-intensity LASER therapy **(Fig. 6)**	• Hot fermentation for 15–20 minutes prior to exercise and stretching • Extracapsular shockwave therapy • Matrix rhythm therapy	Biofeedback	• Blood flow restriction training • Biofeedback	• Blood flow restriction training • Biofeedback

Continued

Continued

Rehabilitation protocol	Phase 1 Early postoperative phase	Phase 2 Late postoperative phase	Phase 3 Early return to function/activity phase	Phase 4 Late return to function/activity phase	Phase 5 Return to sports phase
Duration	0–2 weeks	3–6 weeks	6–8 weeks	8–12 weeks	12 weeks +
Prerequisites for progression	• Minimal pain and no active signs of inflammation • Adherence to precautions	• Adequate healing of surgical repair • Full ROM • Appropriate scapula positioning • Shoulder strength—50–75% of the uninvolved side • Pain-free isometric exercises	• No pain • No signs of active inflammation • Appropriate scapular control • Pain-free activities of daily living • Shoulder strength—90% of the uninvolved side	• No pain • No signs of active inflammation • Appropriate scapular control • Pain-free activities of daily living • Bilateral symmetrical shoulder strength	

General precautions:
- Keep suture site clean and dry
- Avoid sleeping on the operated side in the first two phases
- Avoid excessive activity which may increase inflammation
- Avoid lifting heavy weights in the first two phases

(ADL: activities of daily living; GH: glenohumeral; ROM: range of motion)

CHAPTER 15: Rehabilitation in Arthroscopic Rotator Cuff Repair and Capsular Release...

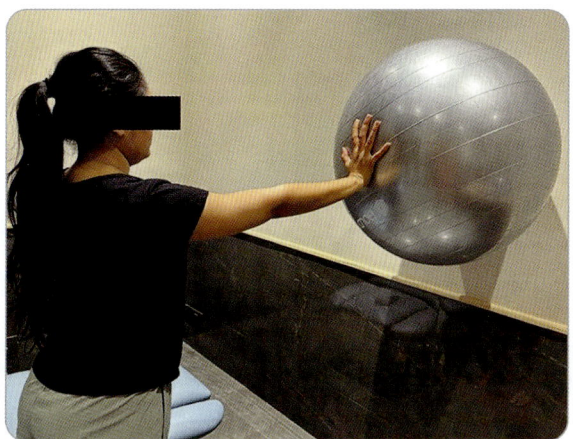

FIG. 1: Shoulder dynamic stabilization exercise.

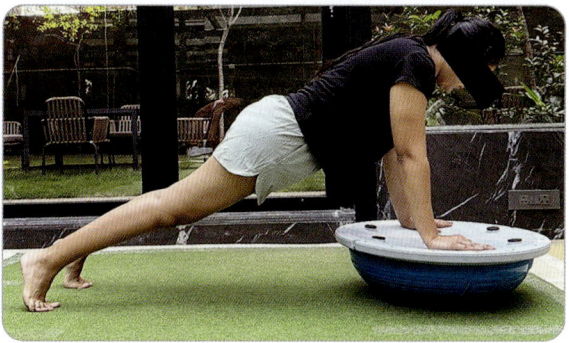

FIG. 2: Shoulder proprioceptive training exercise.

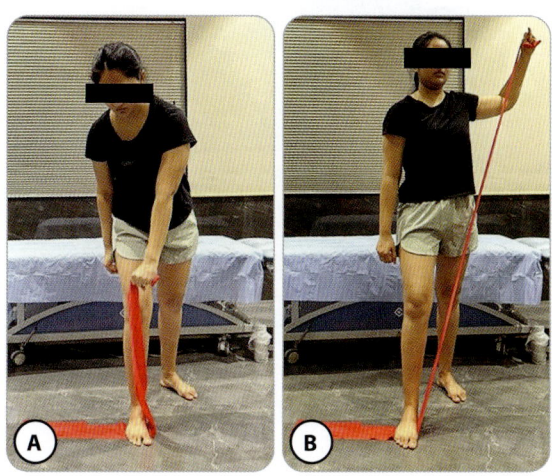

FIGS. 3A AND B: Shoulder proprioceptive neuromuscular facilitation exercise: (A) Start position and (B) end position.

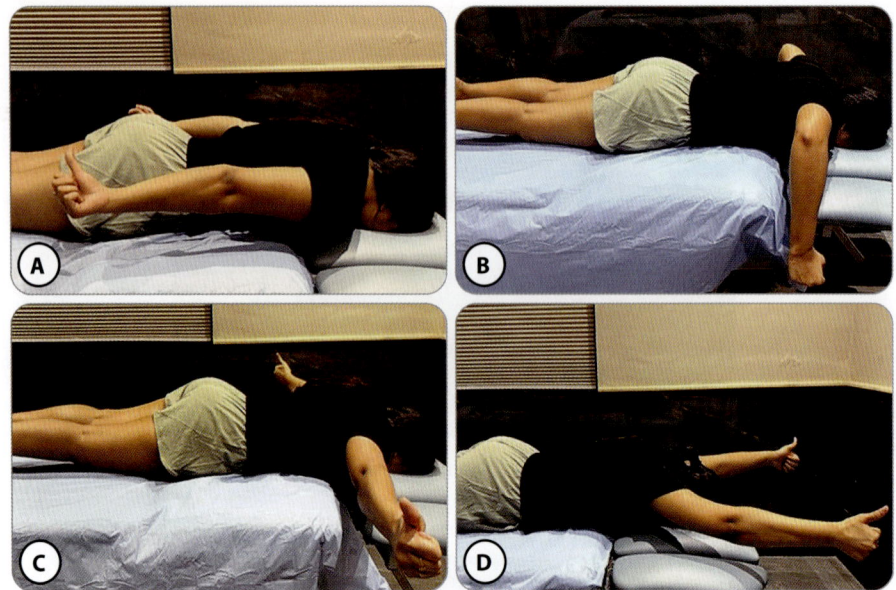

FIGS. 4A TO D: Scapular stabilization exercises: (A) A lifts; (B) Middle trapezius activation; (C) T lifts; and (D) Y lifts.

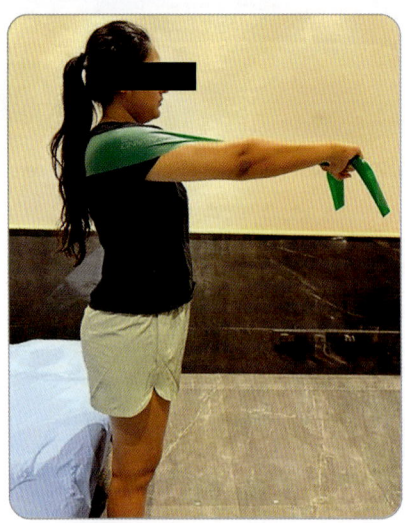

FIG. 5: Serratus anterior strengthening exercise.

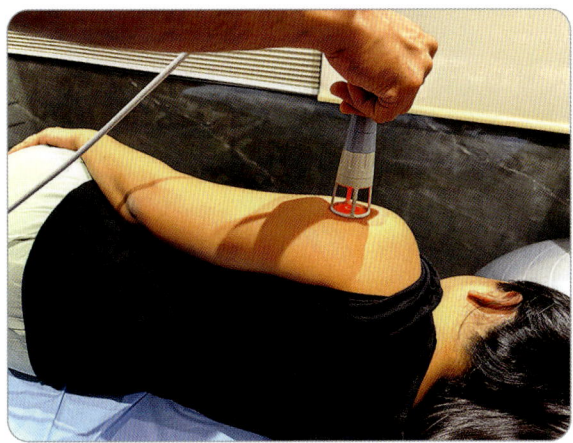

FIG. 6: High-intensity LASER therapy.

SUGGESTED READINGS

1. Akhtar A, Richards J, Monga P. The biomechanics of the rotator cuff in health and disease - A narrative review. J Clin Orthop Trauma. 2021;18:150-6.
2. Sambandam SN, Khanna V, Gul A, Mounasamy V. Rotator cuff tears: An evidence based approach. World J Orthop. 2015;6(11):902-18.
3. Van der Meijden OA, Westgard P, Chandler Z, Gaskill TR, Kokmeyer D, Millett PJ. Rehabilitation after arthroscopic rotator cuff repair: current concepts review and evidence-based guidelines. Int J Sports Phys Ther. 2012;7(2):197-218.
4. Sciarretta FV, Moya D, List K. Current trends in rehabilitation of rotator cuff injuries. SICOT J. 2023;9:14.
5. Fernandes MR. Arthroscopic treatment of adhesive capsulitis of the shoulder with minimum follow up of six years. Acta Ortopédica Bras. 2015;23(2):85-9.
6. Willmore EG, Millar NL, van der Windt D. Post-surgical physiotherapy in frozen shoulder: A review. Shoulder Elb. 2022;14(4):438-51.
7. Galasso O, Mercurio M, Luciano F, Mancuso C, Gasparini G, De Benedetto M, et al. Arthroscopic capsular release for frozen shoulder: when etiology matters. Knee Surg Sport Traumatol Arthrosc. 2023;31(11):5248-54.
8. Puah KL, Salieh MS, Yeo W, Tan AHC. Outcomes of arthroscopic capsular release for the diabetic frozen shoulder in Asian patients. J Orthop Surg. 2018;26(1):2309499018757572.
9. Boutefnouchet T, Jordan R, Bhabra G, Modi C, Saithna A. Comparison of outcomes following arthroscopic capsular release for idiopathic, diabetic and secondary shoulder adhesive capsulitis: A Systematic Review. Orthop Traumatol Surg Res. 2019;105(5):839-46.

Author Publications

1. Sundar MS, Sane RM, Sundaramoorthy R, Ashraf M, Rajan DV. Evaluating transosseous anchorless repair for arthroscopic rotator cuff surgery: a comparative study with double row anchor repair. Clin Shoulder Elb. 2024.
2. Deore S, Patil B, Kale S, Mishra R, Modi R, Mehta N. Management of Neglected Locked Anterior Shoulder Dislocation in the Elderly Population in an Indian Scenario - A Case Report. J Orthop Case Rep. 2024;14(9):87-91.
3. Deore S, Kale S, Chalak A, Ghodke R, Mehta N, Modi R. Trifocal Injury of the Patellar Tendon- An Exceedingly Rare Case Report. J Orthop Case Rep. 2024;14(2):145-9.
4. Deore S N, Kale S, Gunjotikar A, Isaacs N, Achalare A, Das S. An antegrade soft anchor in a retrograde drilling for medial meniscus root repair with high tibial osteotomy: A modified approach to avoid tunnel collision. J Res Prac Mus Sys. 2023;7(3):69-75.
5. Deore S, Kale S, Chalak A, Achalare A, Nalawade V, Doshi SS. Relationship of incidence of anterior cruciate ligament injuries and body-built index somatotype in Indian population. Int J Res Orthop. 2023;9(2):1-7.
6. Kale S, Deore S, Gunjotikar A, Singh S, Ghodke R, Agrawal P. Arthroscopic meniscus repair and augmentation with autologous fibrin clot in Indian population: A 2-year prospective study. J Clin Orthop Trauma. 2022;32:101969.
7. Bhor P, Kale SY, Singh SD, Dhar SB, Garg A, Bukalsaria D. A prospective study of arthroscopic evaluation of patients with chronic shoulder pain. Int J Res Orthop. 2017;3(5):1015-8.
8. Deore S, Patil B, Kale S, Samant P, Ali S. Influence of meniscal repair versus meniscectomy on ACL reconstruction in terms of knee stability and radiological imaging. Int J Orthop Sci. 2017;3(4):853-8.
9. Deore S, Patil B, Samant P, Kale S, Shetty S, Fefar M. Radiological and clinical evaluation amongst types of tibial tunnel widening and choice of graft fixation implants in ACL reconstruction. Int J Orthop Sci. 2017;3(3):1166-72.
10. Date S, Patil S, Gaokar N, Koli V, Solanki M, Pandey P. Functional outcomes of transtibial vs transportal drilling techniques in anterior cruciate ligament reconstruction. Int J Curr Res. 2016;8(10):40556-62.
11. Arora M, Shetty SH, Khedekar RG, Kale S. Over half of badminton players suffer from shoulder pain: Is impingement to blame? J Arth J Surg. 2015;2(1):33-6.
12. Patil B, Arora M, Samant PD, Tripathi M. A case of bilateral posterior medial meniscus root tear: Partial meniscectomy versus pull-out suture repair. J Arth J Surg. 2015;2(1):42-6.

Index

Page number followed by *f* refer to figure, and *t* refer to table.

A

Acromial fracture 91
Acromioclavicular portals 80
Activities of daily living 160
Activity phase 157, 158, 159, 160
Agility ladder drills 148*f*
Anchor placement 102
Anterior capsular release 131*f*
Anterior cruciate ligament 40*f*, 45, 46, 48, 51, 55, 56,
 bundles of 46*f*
 contact lesion on 85*f*
 femoral attachment of 45*f*
 graft with bioscrew 55*f*
 tears on arthroscopy 51*f*
Anterior drawer test 47*f*
Anterior instability 104
 recurrent 111
Anterior labrum 82*f*
Anterior portals 79
 entry 82*f*
Anterior subacromial portal 80
Anterolateral portal 18, 19*f*
 high 18
Anteromedial portal
 accessory 19*f*, 19
 standard 19*f*, 19
Apprehension test 105*f*
Arthroscope and lens 1
Arthroscopic 71*f*, 96, 128
 capsular release, long-term
  rehabilitation of
 examination, sequence of 37
 labral repair 114
 lens 1*f*
 repair, contraindications 112
 rotator cuff repair, long-term
  rehabilitation of 152*t*
 surgeon 137
 surgery, draping for 15

Arthroscopy 1
 diagnostic 50
 surgeon 132
 trolley 7*f*
Augmented techniques 73
Avulsion fractures 107*f*

B

Bag set-up 15*f*
Bankart lesion 109*f*
Barrel length 2
Beach chair position 76, 77, 77*f*
Bear hug test 95*f*
Belly press test 95*f*
Biceps, long head of 82, 82*f*
Bioscrew fixation 56*f*
Bone-patellar tendon-bone graft 23*f*
Bone-tendon-bone 23
 technique, contraindications 25
Bony lesions 91
Bucket handle medial meniscus tear 61*f*, 62*f*

C

Camera console 6*f*
Camera cover 16*f*
Camera head 5*f*
Cannulated screws 124*f*
Capsular release 150
Capsule 38, 39
 labrum complex 117*f*
 lateral 39*f*
 medial 40*f*
 rent 110*f*
 repairing 124*f*
C-arm picture 124*f*
Cartilage lesions 90
Caspari technique 114
Central third quadriceps tendon dissected 30*f*

Index

Clavicular fracture 91
Cold light source 4
Computed tomography 108
Conjoint tendon 130*f*
Contralateral leg, placed 13*f*
Coracoid
   osteotomy 122*f*
   process 79*f*, 130*f*
     drilling holes in 123*f*
     length of 121*f*
     measuring the length of 122*f*
   with oscillating saw 122*f*
Creating portals, technique for 17
Cruciate ligament reconstructions,
     draping for 15
Cryocompression therapy 149*f*
Cuff, assessing retractability of 99*f*
Curette, help of 116*f*
Cutting
   excess suture limbs 119*f*
   sports-specific drills 146*f*
Cyclops formation 51*f*

D

Debris, clearing joint of 57
Deltopectoral incision 120*f*
Diameter 2
Dislocated position 107*f*
Distraction-related complications 89
Draping 13*f*, 14, 77
   steps 16
   video camera 16
Drawer test 106*f*
Drill femoral tunnel 53*f*
Drilling beath pin 54*f*
Drive unit with
   blades 9
   drill attachment 10
Dynamic quadriceps strengthening 148*f*

E

Empty notch 51*f*
Endobutton fixation 56*f*
Entry with dilator 83*f*
ER lag sign 94*f*

F

Femoral anterior cruciate ligament tear 51*f*
Femoral fixation 54, 55*f*
Femoral tunnel 51, 55*f*, 72*f*
   site of 72*f*
Fibrous band connecting 27*f*
Figure-of-4 position 64*f*
Fixation hardware, breakage of 90
Flexed-knee position 11
Footprint 99*f*, 102
   with bare area 100*f*
Freshening meniscus, techniques of 63
Freshening tear 68
Frozen shoulder 126, 150, 151, 157*t*
Function phase 157-160

G

Gastrocnemius 27*f*
Glenohumeral 160
   instrument portal: technique 81
   joint 88*f*
     examination of 87
     intra-articular view of 87*f*
   portals 78
   posterior portal: technique 81
Glenoid 82
   bone, loss of anterior 108*f*
   face of 116*f*
   secondary changes in 107*f*
Gracilis 27*f*
   isolation of 27*f*
   tendon 25
Graft 23, 35*t*
   board 52*f*
   diameter, measurement of 34*f*, 52*f*
   harvesting 28*f*, 30*f*, 50
   length, measurement of 29*f*, 52*f*
   preparation 50
   prepared 52*f*
   pulled 55*f*
   securing 124*f*
   type of 35
Greater tuberosity 92*f*, 107*f*

H

Habermeyer technique 112
Harvested tendon graft 29*f*
Harvesting tendon 33*f*
Healthy bleeding bed, preparing 116*f*
Hill-Sachs lesion 109*f*
Humeral head 82, 82*f*, 130*f*

Index

I

Iliotibial 145
Illumination 4
Impingement test 54
Inferior glenohumeral ligament 128
    mobilizing 115f
Inflamed
    joint 128f
    rotator interval 129f
Infraspinatus 92
Instrument breakage 90
Instrumental portal with shaver 85f
Intercondylar area 39

J

Jobe test 94f
Joint, tight 129f

K

Knee
    agility 146f
    arthroscopy 22f
    diagnostic round 37
    hyperflexion of 53f
    in extension 20f
    joint, examination of 18
    lateral compartment of 41f
    ligament arthroscopic
        long-term rehabilitation of 140t
        surgeries 139
    positioning, draping, and portals 11
    posteromedial compartment of 43f
    proprioception training 147f
Knee scorpion device 67f
Knot tying 119f

L

Labral
    pathology 87f
    repair, three-point 112
Lachman test 47f
Laser therapy, high-intensity 163f
Latarjet reconstruction 120
Lateral compartment 40
Lateral decubitus position 75, 77
Lateral femoral condyl 39f
Lateral meniscus 145
    radial tear of 60f
Lateral position, final setup in 76f
Lateral recess 38, 39f
Lateral subacromial portal 80
Lateral suprapatellar portal 20, 20f
Lateral tibial condyle 39f, 41f
Learning curve 133
    high 134f
Leg-hanging knee position 12f, 13f
Lift off test 95f
Ligamentum mucosum 41f
Light cable 4f

M

Magnetic resonance imaging 48, 62, 96, 97f, 108, 128
Matrix rhythm therapy 149f
McMurray's test 59f, 60f
Medial collateral ligament 28f, 145
    clinical landmark for 64f
Medial compartment 42
Medial coracoid 121f
Medial femoral condyle 40f, 42f, 43f, 71
Medial meniscus 42f, 145
    inside-out repair of 66f
    posterior horn of 42f, 43f
    repair of anterior third of 66f
    tear horizontal tear 61f
Medial recess 39, 40f
Medial suprapatellar portal 19
Medial tibial condyle 40f, 42f, 43f
Meniscal tear patterns 59
Meniscocapsular junction 61f
Meniscus 58
    cutter 9
    tear, repair of horizontal 67
    undersurface of 65f
Mini wall squats 148f
Mitek anchor system 116
Motivational image 134f

N

Nerve lesions 90
Neuromuscular facilitation exercise 161f
Neviaser portal 79f
Notch, roof of 41f

O

One-chip camera 5
Osteotome, curved 122f
Osteotomy 122f

P

Palpation 81
Partial tear 97
   management of 98
Patellar cartilage 23, 37f
Patellofemoral joint 38, 38f
Pectoralis minor 121f
Peek anchor, placing entry owl for 100f
Peroneus
   brevis isolated 33f
   longus 33f
      graft 31
      tendon, incision for 32f
   sheath incised longitudinally 33f
Pes anserinus 28f
Phase return sports phase 152, 153, 157-160
Popliteus insertion 39f
Portal
   related complications 90
   types of 18
Position and jig placement 54f
Position-related complications 89
Posterior cruciate ligament 40f, 43f, 69, 71
   anatomy of 69
   biomechanics of 69
   injuries
      classification of 69
      newer methods of treatment for 73
   reconstruction 71
   repair 73
   sign, double 62f
   tears
      clinical tests for 70
      investigations for diagnosis of 70
      treatment of 70
Posterior portal 78
Posterior subacromial portal 80
Posterolateral portal 21
Posteromedial compartment 42
Posteromedial portal 20
   needle technique for 20f
Probing popliteal hiatus 42f

Q

Quadriceps tendon 29
Quadriceps tendon harvesting instruments 31f

R

Ramp lesions 68
Ramp repair 68f
Ramp tear 61
Range of motion 145, 156, 160
Rehabilitation 139
   in arthroscopic capsular release 151
   in arthroscopic rotator cuff repair 150
   postoperative 73, 137
   protocol 140-160
Release test 105f
Relocation test 105f
Repair techniques 63
Resection 63
   and repair, combined 67
Retropatellar cartilage 37, 38f
Rotation
   external 127f
      weakness in 94f
   internal 127f
Rotator cuff 92, 92f, 101f
   anatomy of 92
   tear 91, 99f, 100f
   etiology of 93
Rotator interval release

S

Scapular
   neck, anterior-inferior 115f
   plane 94f
   stabilization exercises 162f
Semitendinosus 27f
   isolation of 27f
   tendon 25
Serratus anterior strengthening exercise 162f
Shaver 7
   blade 8f
      and burr 9f
      types of 10f
   console handpiece 7f
   foot switch 8f
   handpiece, parts of 8f
Sheath 3
   and obturator 3f
   insertion 81
   insertion of 18
   set up 18f

Shoulder arthroscopy 79*f*
  common portals for 79*f*
Shoulder
  diagnostic round 87
  dynamic stabilization exercise 161*f*
  intra-articular arthroscopic of 82*f*
  movements, restricted 127*f*
  positioning, draping, and portals 75
  proprioceptive training exercise 161*f*
Single leg balance training 147*f*
Skin
  incision 17, 81
  marking 17*f*, 26*f*
Speed test 95*f*
Splitting subscapularis 123*f*
Sports phase 154-156
Step up
  exercise 146*f*
  lateral 147*f*
Sterilizability 3
Stiching rod 82*f*
Stimulate biology 63
Stitching rod, anterosuperior portal 83*f*
Straight-leg
  position 11
  raise 145
Subacromial
  arthroscope portal: technique 85
  bursa 85*f*
  instrument portal: technique 86
  portals 80
  space, examination of 88
Subscapularis 82, 82*f*
Sulcus sign 106*f*
Superior portal 80
Superior recess 37, 37*f*
Superior subacromial portal 80
Supine knee position 12*f*
Supraspinatus 92
Suture
  anchor 119*f*
    insertion of 116*f*
    placing 100*f*
    system 114
  knots 101*f*
  relaying and shuttling 118*f*
  retriever 118*f*

Switching stick and dilator 21*f*
Synovial resector 9
Synovium 37*f*
Synthetic materials 32

T

Tear
  classification 97
  types of 102
Tendinosis, isolation of 27*f*
Tensor fascia lata 145
Tensor fascia latae stretch 146*f*
Teres minor 92
Three-chip camera 6
Tibial anterior cruciate ligament 46*f*
Tibial condyles 56*f*
Tibial fixation 56
Tibial tunnel 52
  site for 72*f*
Torn posterior cruciate ligament 71*f*
Tourniquet placement 14, 14*f*
Transparent relationship, building trust 136
Transverse abdominis 145
Trochlea 37*f*
Tube camera 5

U

Ultrasound 96, 108

V

Valgus stress 64*f*
Vastus medialis obliquus 145
Video camera 5
Video systems 5
Visualization system, components in 6*f*

W

Well-padded 13*f*
Wide graft measured 30*f*

X

Xenon light source 4